Life Music

Lessons Learned at
The University of Catastrophe

Marie Smith

Purple Pen Press
Lombard, Illinois

Cover photographs and design by Steven Smith

Library of Congress Control Number: 2007937902
ISBN: 978-0-6151-6581-3

Purple Pen Press is a division of:
Pen & Bow Productions
P. O. Box 671
Lombard, IL 60148

Printed in the U.S.A.

For Steve and Evelyn,
Thank you for coming with me on the journey
and joining me in the dance.

Contents

The Dance

An Invitation

I enjoy taking long hikes on the Illinois Prairie Path, a trail near my home. If you've jogged along that trail between Elmhurst and Wheaton, you may have seen me. I'm the smiling lady in the purple powerchair cruising along the path. With my service dog Honey trotting beside my chair, I zip along and watch people's reactions to me. I'm pleased to report, the vast majority of people I encounter wave or say hello.

A few people glare at me as if they're thinking, "What are you doing here with us?" Their expressions make perfect sense to me. Seeing me drooling in my powerchair with my head slumped to the side, I'm a stark example of what they don't want to become. I am what many people fear. So, I have compassion for them. Still, the scowls are the exception. Like I said before, most people smile and wave. Some even stop and chat.

But, I often wonder as the friendly cyclists and joggers pass me on the path, do they realize I used to ride a bike, play soccer, cross country ski, snowshoe, snorkel and swim? Or do they assume I was always cruising through

v

life on a powerchair. Do they assume I grew up different from them, going to special schools, riding a special bus? Perhaps they assume growing up as a special needs kid somehow prepared me for life as the drooling lady in the purple powerchair who sometimes talks funny.

The truth is, nothing in my past prepared me for life inside this body. I had the opportunity to study *Pain and Suffering, Disability and You,* and *Advanced Studies in Wheelchair Maintenance,* in college. But, I dropped those classes and focused my attention on far more important things: beer, beer, hangovers and beer.

I grew up a fairly regular kid. Apart from my overwhelming addiction to my cello and life threatening allergy to homework, I was a typical child. Absolutely nothing I experienced in the first 27 years of my life prepared me for what I was about to endure.

When I was 27, I went to bed April 14th, 1997 an ordinary wife and mother of a six-year-old daughter. That night I curled up in bed with my book, and my cat, and I fell asleep. I woke up the next morning blind and in agony.

Ever have a leg cramp wake you up at night? Remember you leapt out of bed and frantically stretched your calf trying to get rid of the charley horse? Remember how much that hurt? OK, now imagine if that pain was in your eye.

I had a charley horse in my eye muscle and no way to stretch it. It felt like an unseen hand jammed a red hot corkscrew in my right eye. The pain lasted over a year. It took 14 months and 17 doctors to diagnose me with myasthenia gravis. MG is a rare neuromuscular disease. It is progressive, incurable and sometimes fatal.

I remember moving easily, but now I feel like I lurch through invisible tar. Inside, I'm full of life and energy. Outside, my body is worn out and I feel old beyond my years. Myasthenia gravis makes it difficult for me to see, chew, swallow, hold up my head, sit upright, smile, speak, close my jaw, walk, move my arms, dress myself, feed myself, brush my hair, brush my teeth, breathe and move. Due to medication side effects I also struggle to think clearly, remember things and communicate. I also drool from the medicine.

This is my reality, and I am not special, extraordinary, or especially gifted to handle this catastrophe. What I am is a woman up a creek without a paddle.

Everyone spends part of their lives up a creek without a paddle. No one is exempt from the journey. Some people get wet for a little while and then find their way to shore again. They shake themselves off, go on with their lives, and laugh about it for years.

Others spend more time up a creek without a paddle. They sink and swim, float and dog paddle through rapids and over waterfalls. They get banged up on rocks and bitten by snapping turtles and alligators. When the creek bends, and they finally escape, there is no thought of shaking themselves off and going on with life. There is just a long time lying on the shore, stunned to still be alive. Life will never be the same again. They are forever marked by scars the white water rapids left behind.

And then there are people like me. For me, being up Nightmare Creek without a paddle is normal. Right now

I'm bumping through yet another white water rapids. I started a powerful MG treatment three weeks ago. My disease is so out of control my neurologist referred me to oncology for treatment. As I'm typing this, my hair is falling out from chemotherapy. My hair keeps landing on the computer keyboard and tangling around my fingers. Losing my hair is making me laugh, and cry, and laugh again. I have no idea if the chemotherapy will help me.

Floating along Nightmare Creek, bouncing through rapids and careening down waterfalls, I'm surprised by how often the journey fascinates me. No, I didn't sign up. If my doctor offered me a cure tomorrow, I'd take it. However, life up Nightmare Creek is amazing to me. It's the greatest physical, intellectual, and spiritual challenge of my life.

Just how do you lose your physical abilities without losing your sense of self? How do you graciously let go of the use of your own body? How do you keep your faith? Your sanity? How do you keep from getting so depressed you drink, use drugs, or take your life? Where do you find the strength to face another day?

There is no map or specially trained guide to help you along the way. Trust me, I've looked. No one asked my opinion before I was unceremoniously dumped in Nightmare Creek. So, how am I supposed to live like… this?

I have no idea. But, the journey so far has been worth every bump, bruise, and scar. I have many scars on my body and even more on my soul. So, I float along assuming the rest of the trip will be worth it, too. It's been an amazing adventure and I'd love to tell you what I've amazing adventure and I'd love to tell you what I've learned.

I've left out my husband and daughter's reactions. This journey has been tough on all three of us. Steve and Evelyn's thoughts and feelings are their stories to tell, not mine. However, I will tell you what I've discovered. While I tread water, I invite you to grab yourself a snack, and have a seat on that flat rock by the water's edge, so we can celebrate life together.

The Journey

Orange on Blue
(for Lee)

While powerchair cruising on the Illinois Prairie Path last Friday afternoon, I looked up and saw a maple tree. Dressed in fiery orange for autumn, the tree stretched its branches toward a cloudless Illinois blue sky. A gentle breeze fluttered the leaves and the tree swayed in the warm October sun. I stopped, told Honey to lie down, and just marveled at the tree. Seeing orange leaves against a pure blue sky, I burst into tears at the wonder of it. Under that tree, I celebrated having eyes that see.

In 1997, the first thing myasthenia gravis took from me was my eyesight. Overnight, I lost half of my sight and gradually lost more. Within months, I was almost completely blind. My eyes became so sensitive to light, a birthday candle made me squint. I wore dark green glasses that only let 1% light through them. Through my protective lenses the world was shadowy green.

Before April 1997, the closest I came to blindness was a trust walk at summer camp. Blindfolded and lead by another kid down a wooded trail, I trusted my friend to keep me from stumbling. But, that was just a game. When it was over, I took off the blindfold and went back to being my sighted self. In April 1997, my sighted self vanished and I had no idea how to cope.

Like I said before, I was 27 when I got sick. The sum total of my life experiences added up to exactly diddlysquat. When my sight went haywire, I calmly assessed the situation and came up with a rational plan of action. Wait. No, I didn't. I completely freaked! Of course I freaked. I mean, what would you do? I woke up with a blind woman's eyes in my skull and doctors had no idea what was wrong with me.

At first, they thought I might have a brain tumor. When the MRI came back normal, I became a medical ping-pong ball and bounced from one eye specialist to another. Dr. One referred me to Dr. Two. Dr. Two referred me to Dr. Three, and on it went. I had appointments with 16 eye specialists, ate painkillers like candy, and could barely see.

Losing my eyesight made the most basic tasks amazingly hard. Setting the dishwasher knob, tying my shoes, sorting laundry, cooking dinner, even making a cup of tea were almost impossible. Doctors shined bright lights in my sensitive eyes, but didn't help me function. When I burned dinner, because I couldn't see the numbers on my kitchen timer, I knew I needed help. I couldn't wait for a diagnosis. Not knowing where else to turn, I called The Chicago Lighthouse for the Blind and Visually Impaired.

At the Chicago Lighthouse, I met Lee Logan. She works in the Strickfaden Assistive Devices Store selling adaptive equipment. Though I was confused and scared, Lee welcomed me into the store and showed me many different types of adaptive equipment.

I never knew so many gadgets existed. Talking microwaves. Talking watches. Talking bathroom scales. Know what? You need a lot of self confidence to step on a scale and hear your weight announced in a cheerful electronic voice. I was afraid the scale would say, "Ouch! Lose some weight, tubby!" So, I didn't step on the scale. I did get a talking wristwatch, a large print kitchen timer, and a new friend.

Visually impaired herself, Lee knows a lot about adapting to life with less eyesight. She taught me the basic rules. If print is too small to see, find some way to make it bigger so you can see it. Use contrasting colors to help you see things. Put Velcro on the dishwasher knob to help you run the dishwasher by touch. And most importantly, get a white cane and learn to use it.

I got a white cane and swept it in front of me like a broom. I still crashed into chairs and walls. Lee taught me how to use a cane to walk in a straight line. She taught me how to cross a street when I couldn't see the traffic lights or the crosswalk. With my cane I learned to sense what was around me. Gravel. Grass. Carpet. Tile. Snow. Sand. My cane also bumped into obstacles before I did. It went down a step or a curb before I fell. I remember my cane made a swishing sound as I walked through leaves on the sidewalk, stirring the fallen leaves into perfume.

Losing my eyesight taught me to pay more attention to my other senses. It's a myth that people with visual impairments have super hearing. They just use their hearing differently. For example, shut your eyes and drop a quarter and a dime on a hard floor. Do it over and over until you can hear the difference between the coins. If you get really good at it, you can hear change land on the ground and say, "You dropped 53¢." I never got good at it, but I did learn to use my ears.

Since I couldn't see people approaching, I learned to recognize my friends by their footsteps. Even though I could tell who people were before they spoke, they always announced themselves. This secretly amused me.

Once I could get around safely with my cane, and learned to use my hearing to help me, I grew frustrated. Bet you thought I was going to say grateful. Nope. Frustrated. I was frustrated by all of the things I could no longer do. Watch TV. Watch the birds at the bird feeders in my yard. Read. As time went on and my sight didn't improve, I felt abandoned and angry. I grew bitter and hopeless. Then Lee introduced me to Braille.

Braille is essentially a code based on six raised dots in various combinations to represent letters. It took a few weeks of practice to memorize the letters, but it wasn't as hard to learn as I thought it would be. Actually, it was fun.

At first, the book had raised letters beside the Braille dots. I felt the letter A, and learned which dot represented A. Then I did the same for the letter B, and C, and so on. The first word I read in Braille was cab. The first sentence I read in Braille was, "Abe bagged a bad cabbage." I laughed when I read it. Within days, the dots began to feel like letters. Soon, I was reading again.

Learning to read Braille opened my mind to new possibilities. I was in my backyard when I heard chickadees calling. No, I couldn't see the birds in my yard anymore, but I could hear them. I learned to recognize my favorite birds by their calls.

A year after I lost my sight, I sat on a bench beside a blooming lilac bush and listened to a chorus of birds. That's when I realized I was still able to enjoy life. Not despite losing my sight. I was still able to enjoy life because I was alive and surrounded by the beauty of spring.

Not being able to see allowed me to enjoy spring a new way. Smelling lilacs, and hearing robins, American cardinals, song sparrows, house wrens, and chickadees, I knew I hadn't lost sight of the world. I just experienced it in new ways. Though I lost my eyesight, I didn't lose my vision.

Up until that time in my life, I learned about the world with my eyes first and other senses later. Losing my sight forced me to pay more attention to my other four senses. To my surprise, I gradually found myself delighted by the change.

Touching the cat I couldn't see made me appreciate the softness of her fur, and the vibrations I felt when she purred. I couldn't see the mint growing in my garden, but I could smell it when the plants brushed my leg. Chocolate still tastes better with my eyes closed. And I've known since I was small that my cello sounds best when I close my eyes and just listen to him sing. After spending a year with limited eyesight, I knew I could still enjoy life even if I never got my sight back.

If it hadn't been for the pain in my right eye, I would have given up going to doctors and simply accepted life behind dark green glasses. But, I was in pain. In the spring of 1998, the pain in my eye increased beyond painkillers. Every night REM sleep made me sit up in bed and scream at the top of my lungs. It felt like my eyeball was going to pop like a balloon. It hurt so much suicide crossed my mind.

For a year I went to eye specialists, always hoping for relief that never came. So, in early June of 1998, I gave up on eye doctors. I could live without eye sight. The pain had to stop. Using a high powered magnifying glass I searched for pain relief in the phone book. In the yellow pages, I found an entry in big red letters for an anesthesiologist. It was the only ad large enough for me to read. So, I picked up the phone and called Dr. 17.

At my first appointment, Dr. 17 did something so radical none of the other 16 specialists even thought of doing it. He got a book off the shelf and then looked up my symptoms. The doctor said he thought I might have a rare neuromuscular disease. "It's so rare, I've never actually seen it before."

After running a test at the hospital the next day, Dr. 17 diagnosed me with myasthenia gravis. I remember thinking, "It has a name. I'm not crazy. It has a name." Relief and dread washed over me at the same time.

Once he had a diagnosis, Dr. 17 opened his book again. The book told him to write me a prescription for a drug called Mestinon. Mestinon is the first drug used to treat myasthenia gravis. I won't bore you with the details of how Mestinon works. Let me just say that Mestinon is a drug that helps muscles and nerves communicate better.

At home I took one Mestinon tablet. Within half an hour, the muscle spasm in my eye finally disappeared. For the first time in 14 months, I wasn't in pain. My eyes were no longer sensitive to light. I took off the green glasses and saw the world in blurry colors. I remember crying for a totally different reason.

I blinked a few times, and my sight returned as if nothing had ever happened to me. It was amazing! I looked into my husband's eyes. I hadn't seen Steve in over a year. I looked at my little daughter's face and saw Evelyn smile at me.

Everything I saw made me wild with joy. Stars. The moon. I treasured seeing birds again and flowers in my garden. Squirrels. Butterflies. Wood paneling. Cat hair on the carpet. Ketchup stains on Evelyn's pink shirt. If I could see it, it was worth celebrating.

That was many years ago. Has the joy worn off? Do I take my eyes for granted? Of course I do. That's why the sight of that beautiful maple tree made me cry on Friday. I felt such shame as I watched the orange leaves flutter to the ground. All the time I pass beautiful things and don't notice. Too often I forget to pause and treasure what my eyes see.

But every once in a while, I remember where I've been, and I look at this world anew. I stop and cherish seeing frost sparkle on the grass. A friend's smile. A blue heron in flight. Dew on an orb spider web. Snowcapped mountains in Colorado. And vivid orange maple leaves singing a duet with an Illinois clear blue sky.

The University of Catastrophe

Myasthenia gravis is Greek and Latin for *grave muscle weakness*. About 36,000 Americans have this rare disease. To put that in perspective, more than 36,000 Americans live in my hometown. Somehow I won the lottery in reverse and ended up with MG.

Even though I didn't want to, I learned all I could about the disease. Since the medical explanation uses imaginary words like neurotransmitter, acetylcholine receptor, anti-acetylcholine receptor antibody, and the like, I'm going to simplify things.

If you want to research myasthenia gravis in depth, be my guest. Surf the web and look it up. Me? I've read enough medical jargon to know I hate reading medical jargon. I'd much rather explain the effects of MG instead of discussing the technical aspects. In the end, that's what matters anyway.

To help you understand myasthenia gravis, I want you to imagine a telephone. No, not your cell phone. Think back to the olden days. Telephones used to have a base, a receiver and a curly cord between the two. Picture that kind of phone in your mind. The phone I'm imagining is a lovely 1970's blinding orange, but yours can be any color.

When you use a telephone, the sound comes from the base, travels up the curly cord, into the receiver. Your body works in a similar way. Your brain says to walk, the information travels through your nerves to the appropriate muscles, and you walk. But, it doesn't always work that way.

Imagine if you were talking on the phone and the little plastic doohickey that connects the curly cord to the receiver broke. Could you hear your friend anymore? No, because the junction between the curly cord and the receiver broke. Even if your friend was still talking, you wouldn't hear a word.

Myasthenia gravis symptoms happen because of an interrupt between nerve cells and muscle cells. In the junction where nerve cells tell muscle cells to move, there's an interrupt inside my body. Just like with a broken telephone cord, signals don't get through from my brain, even though my brain is still sending a signal. My muscles don't always realize they're supposed to move. MG turns me into a living rag doll.

MG is a disease of the nerve/muscle junction. Did you know you had a nerve/muscle junction? Me neither. Then again, I didn't know I had a lot of body parts until 1998. In preschool, I learned to point to my head, shoulders, knees and toes. No one asked me to point to my manubrium. The fact I can point to mine irritates me to no end.

Where did I get my medical knowledge? I'm glad you asked. I learned all this at The University of Catastrophe. I'd like to graduate from The University of Catastrophe since I already have my master's degree in medical mayhem. But, I can't seem to get the dean to pin down a date for graduation. So, I'm still enrolled against my will at The University of Catastrophe.

Right now I'm taking a class called *Chemotherapy and You*. In case you were wondering, this class really sucks. We're studying two books. One book is called *Puking: Not Just For Hangovers Anymore*. The other book is called *Hats, Turbans, Scarves, and Wigs: You Can Wear Them*. This book is full of illustrations of lovely head coverings that I'd wear all the time. If I lived alone on an island and only if it was dark.

There are many different majors at The University of Catastrophe, but they all have two things in common. No one signs up for classes on purpose and all courses of study suck.

During orientation at a normal university, you're given an overview of what to expect. Orientation at The University of Catastrophe is nothing like that. There is no overview, or newcomer's information packet. You just suddenly find yourself enrolled with a major you didn't chose. You look around at your classmates and wonder, "How did I end up here?"

If you are anything like me, your first reaction is shocked disbelief. I didn't take the prerequisite courses and I don't belong in this class. The assignments are too hard and I don't have the right books. The exams are impossible. I don't even know why I'm here.

Wait! I know! There must be some kind of mistake on my schedule. Why didn't I think of that before? I'll head down to the guidance counseling office and get this cleared right up.

Trot down the hall to the guidance counseling office. Push open a creaky door. What was that? Was that a pigeon flying around? How come there are dusty broken chairs in the counseling office? Doesn't anyone work here? Hello! Can I get some help, please? What's going on?

That's when I discovered there is no mercy at The University of Catastrophe. No one cares if I'm unprepared for class. I'm expected to participate anyway, since dropping classes is against school policy. There is no honor code, because cheating isn't possible. No study guides. No syllabi. No *Cliff's Notes*. No wise professors to guide me. The University of Catastrophe is the toughest school on earth. Everything I thought I knew about life faded into dust the day I enrolled.

During my years as a University of Catastrophe student, I've learned many things. I've discovered not everyone laughs at the same things. A movie I think is hilarious might not make you grin. Sitting in the sunshine drinking tea, and then playing cello duets with a friend, is my idea of a perfect afternoon. You might rather be fishing. Or racing cars. Or painting. Or baking cupcakes with your kids. Not everyone enjoys the same things. But, chances are, what makes you cry will make me cry, too. Trouble bridges gaps between people. We find out we're more alike than we thought, and a shared trouble can bond people closer than family.

Unfortunately, when trouble comes my first instinct is to hide. I pretend I'm doing fine and I don't need any help. Before I ended up at The University of Catastrophe, I liked helping people. If someone asked me to reach a box of rice on a shelf, I was glad to get it. Helping people made me feel useful and happy.

However, asking for help made me feel useless and unhappy. I valued my independence and ability to look after myself. That all changed when I ended up at The University of Catastrophe. Suddenly, I couldn't look after myself and that bothered me.

Chemotherapy is changing how my mind works. I find I have difficulty controlling my emotions. If something isn't where I expect it to be, I meltdown and cry like a toddler. This is bad enough in my kitchen, but in the grocery store when I can't find the right brand of tea, it's unbearable. I know in my mind that my reaction is irrational, but that doesn't stop the tears. Chemotherapy scrambles my brain like an egg.

I can do two things to solve this problem. I can decide not to go grocery shopping anymore. It's too stressful, too embarrassing, and I can't handle it. I can stay at home and isolate from the world. Or, I can ask someone on staff for help.

Since I've been shopping at the same little market for the past 18 years, everyone recognizes me and my service dog, Honey. I cruise in on my powerchair and ask someone to help me shop. Someone is always glad to help me find the bananas, vanilla yogurt, mango green tea, or chocolate bars. So, I can go shopping, even when chemo rubs my emotions raw. All I have to do is ask for help and everything is OK.

Asking for help is still hard for me, but I'm getting better at it. I was visiting friends recently and my arm muscles weakened during dinner. I simply couldn't move my spoon from my plate to my mouth anymore. Horrified, I sat there looking at my limp hands. What do I do? I'm a guest and I can't feed myself! I felt odd and out of place. Stomach growling, I looked at my ravioli and meatballs. What do I do?

Everyone at the table noticed I was having trouble. I felt embarrassed. Hannah asked, "Do you need some help?"

I was almost too embarrassed to say yes. I almost said I wasn't hungry. Instead, I took a deep breath and admitted I couldn't move my arms. Hannah picked up her dinner and sat beside me. My friend took my spoon from me and helped me finish dinner. She fed me, and herself, conversation continued and the world didn't come to an end.

While sitting beside my friend, I was suddenly aware Hannah was glad to help me. Not upset or angry. Just glad to help a friend who needed help. Had I pretended I wasn't hungry anymore, I would have denied Hannah the chance to be helpful. I would have lost an opportunity to grow closer to my friend. Instead I enjoyed my ravioli, and the loving company of a friend, all at the same time.

Help: You Can Ask For It and *Help: You Can Accept It*, were two of the toughest classes I took at The University of Catastrophe. But, the lessons were worth learning.

When I ask for help, I'm not being useless. I'm just letting someone else be helpful. Most people like being helpful, so it works out well for both of us. When I show my weakness, I allow someone else to use their strength. Like my grapevine grows by sending out fragile tendrils, asking for help connects me to others and it connects others to me. Then we both grow stronger and enjoy life together.

Thym... What?

Now you would think myasthenia gravis would be enough to study at The University of Catastrophe. But, you'd be wrong. A few days after I was diagnosed with MG, I returned to Dr. 17's office for a follow up appointment. I arrived at his office without sunglasses or a white cane. Remembering that is making me smile.

Thanks to Dr. 17's help, I could see and I wasn't hurting anymore. I thought every problem was solved thanks to the wonder drug Mestinon. At my appointment, Dr. 17 held out a red pen. "One pen or two?"

I saw one. Since I'd hardly seen anything for 14 months, I was quite excited by that. He bumped my knee with a round mallet and said everything was fine. I was relieved.

Then Dr. 17 got a serious look on his face. "Mrs. Smith, I've been reading up on MG. It turns out, myasthenia gravis can be a paraneoplastic disorder."

Paraneoplastic, really? That's what I suspected all along. Wow doc! That information helped tremendously.

Wait. No, it didn't!

I think I speak for just about everyone when I say, "Huh?" Does paraneoplastic recycle? Does it go in the green bin or the blue bin? I had no idea what he was talking about. To me, it sounded like a bunch of Pig Latin backwards. So, I just sat there nodding.

Dr. 17 said, "You need a chest MRI to scan your thymus gland."

OK, that got my attention. Chest MRI, I understood that part. But thymus gland? I can point to my elbow. I can point to my big toe. I can find my ears. But, what in the world is a thymus gland? You know, I could have lived the rest of my life in blissful ignorance. Except, I was forced to attend The University of Catastrophe and required to take *Thymus Glands: You Have One, Too.*

I was about to ask a question, when Dr. 17 patted my shoulder and gently said, "Don't worry."

Now, true or false. Patting my shoulder and saying, "Don't worry," will calm me right down? True. *Buzz!* I'm sorry; your answer is incorrect! As soon as I'm told not to worry, I worry. Worry wanders around my guts until she finds her daughter Panic, and together Worry and Panic go hunting for Alarm. Don't worry? Right. Like that was gonna happen. I had absolutely no clue what Dr. 17 was talking about and already I was flying toward a panic attack at warp speed.

Patting my shoulder again, Dr. 17 added, "Thymoma is extremely rare."

Is it me, or does thymoma sound like some kind of spicy chicken casserole with onions and peppers? Mmm, pass me more of that thymoma. I still had no idea what the doctor was talking about, but I assumed he wasn't inviting me to dinner. So, I very wisely asked, "Thym... what?"

"Thymoma." With a soft sigh, Dr. 17 said, "Myasthenia gravis symptoms are rarely a warning sign of thymus gland cancer, Mrs. Smith. Thymomas happen mostly to older people and I don't think you have a tumor. We just need an MRI of your chest as a precaution. So, don't worry."

OK. Now that I've heard the word cancer, I'm supposed to *not* worry? Excuse me? What planet is this doctor from? Jupiter? I suppose on Jupiter it might be possible for an emotional, artsy-fartsy, passionate cellist like me not to worry. Here on planet earth, worry was a given.

Obviously, I was worried. Trying to come to terms with a chronic illness is tough. Add possible cancer and I was a wreck. Life's rollercoaster was headed up a big hill. I heard the chains clanking. Would it flatten out? Or was I about to fall?

The University of Catastrophe classes, *Test Results: You Can Wait For Them* and *Test Results II: The Negative Side of Positive*, were informative. While I waited to find out if I had a thymoma, I realized I'd had test results go both ways. Negative for a brain tumor. Positive for MG. Was this a comfort? No way! When I was diagnosed with MG, I found out I wasn't invincible and bad things could happen to me. Not to neighbors, or strangers, but to me. Knowing that made worry and fear stronger. I couldn't sleep. All I could think about was the MRI.

Eleven days later, I got the MRI results. They showed a small thymoma tumor. The radiologist recommended a CT scan to confirm the findings. Five days before my 29th birthday, I had the CT scan. It showed a larger tumor than the MRI did. The day after my birthday,

I met with a surgeon. At the surgeon's request, I had a second CT scan. It found the same 4x3x2 cm tumor in the top of my thymus gland.

The tumor was directly under the notch in my breastbone, extending into my throat. The radiologist couldn't tell if the cancer had spread. Everything I worried about came true. To make matters worse, my diseased thymus gland grew itself around my aorta twice. I needed a median sternotomy. A surgeon was going to split my sternum through my notch to remove the tumor. The planned incision was more radical than open heart surgery.

A few days before surgery, an OR nurse called me and said, "I have to warn you, it will be easier to die than survive surgery. I'm calling to make sure you have your affairs in order."

I was 29! I didn't know which affairs I was supposed to have in order. After talking to the nurse, I worried my daughter would grow up without her mother. What if I do survive surgery? How much will it hurt? What if I can't play my cello anymore? What if...

Worrying handcuffs me to a chain of what if's. What if this happened? What if that happened? I can go on asking, "what if," forever. Trust me. I'm good at worrying. For most of my life, if I was awake I was worried about something. With my vivid imagination, I can cook up terrifying scenarios and scare myself senseless.

For years I chided myself for worrying. Jesus taught, "No one ever added a moment to their life by worrying." I've heard worrying can subtract life from your years. Worrying doesn't fix anything. Worry is... Enough!

I know. I know. But, knowledge doesn't stop my thundering heart, racing mind and sweating palms. Did you know I am fully capable of worrying that I worry too much?

Knowledge didn't turn off the worry switch. It just made me feel stupid for worrying and worried I'd always be that way. Kicking myself doesn't help and life has beaten me up enough already. So, instead of putting myself down for worrying, I've decided to accept being a worrywart.

When life hits the fan I automatically duck for cover and worry about what's coming next. Worry is a reflex for me. If I get tree pollen in my nose, I sneeze. If a surgeon talks about cracking my chest with a bone saw, for some odd reason, I worry. Knowing I have a serious, incurable disease makes me worry about my future. That's how I'm wired. Except for a lobotomy rerouting my wiring, I have to live with worry.

Wait. A lobotomy would require another surgery to worry about. Scratch that. A lobotomy is definitely out.

It took a few years, but I did find a way to make worry easier to live with. Instead of pushing worry away, I let worry in.

I imagined my life was like a giant table in a banquet hall. Since Worry crashed every party, I might as well put her on the guest list. So, I gave Worry a seat at my life's table. Worry, her lover Fear, and their children Alarm and Panic, sat down together and started making a fuss. I listened to them for a moment, and then chose where I would sit.

I sat down at the other end of the table, between Faith and Courage, across from Hope, Joy, and their sister

Laughter. Because of where I'm sitting, to hear Worry's comments and play the what if game, I have to ignore Faith and Courage, Hope, Joy and Laughter.

Faith reminds me to believe everything will turn out OK, even if the evidence appears otherwise. Courage reminds me that feeling terrified, but doing the right thing anyway, is the antidote to Fear's paralyzing stings. Hope whispers of the trials in my past I've survived and encourages me to believe I'll continue being strong. Joy wiggles happily, utterly contented in the smallest things. A sunset. A purring cat. A child's kiss. And Laughter laughs whenever Joy wiggles. The chair where I sit is called Peace. It's hard to worry when you're sitting in Peace.

Worry is still with me constantly and I do sometimes play the what if game. Only now when I start playing, Laughter giggles until I laugh at myself for falling into the same old trap. Joy shows me something simple to remind me to wonder. A ladybug crawling on a blade of grass. Sunlight on a pond. A downy woodpecker drumming on a pear tree. Slowly, I shift my attention away from Worry and go back to my seat at the banquet table. Love and Family are waiting for me. Friendship smiles and holds my hand. I return to the seat of Peace and feel contented.

As I'm typing this, my eyelashes are falling out. I blinked and three of them landed on my glasses and nose. I could worry now. What if I lose more eyelashes? What if someone stares at me because my eyebrows look like a lunatic plucked them? I could play the what if game right now. But, I won't.

Instead, I'm laughing, because my eyebrows and eyelashes are falling out! How absurd and screwy is that? I'm joyful because my cat is purring behind my head and my service dog is snoozing with her chin on my thigh. My dog and cat remind me I'm loved by many and not because I have long beautiful eyelashes and perfect eyebrows. I'm loved heart to heart and that has nothing to do with eyebrows and eyelashes.

Sitting here, I'm hopeful, because I'm bald and the world didn't come to an end. I'm feeling courageous, because I'm fighting for my life. There is quiet dignity in that fight. And I still have faith that I'll be fully alive until my last breath, whenever it comes. In this, I find the peace to face tomorrow.

The Land of the Living
(For Nada)

Every spring daffodils and tulips bloom in my back-yard. A few pink and purple hyacinths fill my garden with their lovely scent. I planted my garden in October 1998, just three months after surgery. I could say, "I'll never forget the day I had surgery," but I'd be lying. The truth is, I remember very little.

I arrived at the hospital, filled out paperwork, said the hardest goodbye of my life to my husband, and followed a nurse into a busy room. After I put on a hospital gown, hands guided me and I stretched out on a gurney. I got an IV in my arm and watched as a man taped the IV in place. I sat up and got a spinal catheter in my back for pain relief after surgery. It didn't hurt as much as I thought it would and I'm a needle fearing coward.

Then the anesthesiologist said something about medication to help me relax. Relaxing sounded like a good idea. I watched her hands moving, putting a needle in the IV line. Then I looked at a hideous yellow-green wall. The wall clock said it was a little after six in the morning.

I blinked.

I looked at a hideous yellow-green wall. The wall clock said it was a little after five in the evening. Hands touched my arms and face. Voices chattered words I couldn't comprehend. "Mrs. Smith. Mrs. Smith?"

Who is Mrs. Smith? Where is Mrs. Smith. For that matter, what is a Mrs. Smith?

"C'mon. It's time to wake up. Surgery is over. You did great."

I did what? Surgery is over? How can that be? It's only been a second. I turned my head a millimeter to the left. Apparently, that little head bob was the cue for the gorilla on my chest to dance. I'm not kidding. Right under my chin an invisible 500 pound gorilla – wearing extra sharp golf cleats – danced! Now, *that* woke me up! The pressure directly under my chin stunned me. I could hardly breathe. The pain was just off the scale. Not surprising, considering for the past nine and a half hours my entire rib cage was ripped in two down the center. Hand me the bone saw. Anyone seen my rib spreader? Sorry, I think I left it hanging on my barbecue grill.

There are no words to fully describe the pain of a median sternotomy and I know why. When the English language was in its infancy, and some poor dude got a battle axe imbedded in his chest, he died before he had a chance to cry out. He certainly didn't invent a new word on his way to a dirt nap. Whack! Dead. Meanwhile, I clung to life.

While this gorilla danced on my chest, I opened my eyes and wanted to say something, but all I managed was a groan. I stayed in that room with the ugly yellow-green paint for a minute. Or fifteen hours. Time was all the same to me. So, I can't say I remember August 21, 1998. But, I'm forever marked by the seven inch scar on my chest, and memories from the fight to recover. It was so difficult, my life is divided into before surgery and after.

Anyone who attends The University of Catastrophe is required to take *Nightmares: You Will Have Them*. Difficult situations leave painful memories in their wake. We all have rotten memories. Mine are alphabetized and carefully labeled in an archive in my mind. When I least expect it, a rotten memory DVD pops into the player in my brain and I find myself reliving one of my least happy times. Whenever this happens, I wish I had an internal delete key. But, I don't. Sometimes I feel doomed to remember what I want to forget.

When I first got sick, my whole life felt like I was riding a conveyer belt. Take these pills. This might be uncomfortable. See this doctor. Lie still. We need a blood sample. Cough. You need a chest x-ray. Come back in a month. You need an MRI. Big stick, take a deep breath. Can I see your insurance card? I'm looking at your repeat CT scan and I'm seeing a tumor. You have an appointment at 2:30 on Friday. Don't eat or drink anything after midnight. I'm putting medicine in your IV. On a scale of one to ten, how much pain are you in right now? You need another IV. Here's your prescription. Take these pills every morning before breakfast. You have a co-pay of. . .

On and on the conveyer belt went, taking me where I never wanted to go. The only way to survive was to stuff all emotions in a box marked later. In a numb daze, I followed the nurse into that yellow-green room. Knowing full well in less than two hours a surgeon was going to carve me like a roast, I still went into that room. If I felt terrified, I couldn't have done it. That morning, I had to ride the medical conveyer belt and there was no room for fear. Fear would have to wait until later. Much later, it turned out.

The Later Box remained in the basement of my soul until all the emotions I'd pushed away came back in a rushing wave in May 2005. My MG symptoms were so severe, my doctor wondered if my thymoma grew back. He ordered a CT scan.

Looking at my chart, the technician asked, "Oh, I see you had a CT of your chest in 1998. What was the result?"

Trembling in my powerchair, I said, "I had surgery to remove a thymoma tumor that extended into my throat."

The technician's eyes widened. "Wow. Let's hope the results are better this time."

I whispered, "They have to be better." While lying on my back in the CT scanner with my arms behind my head and an IV taped to my left hand, the Later Box blew open like a bomb. As tears rolled down my face, I remembered. . . everything.

I remembered the day after surgery, when my heart became unstable and I nearly died. The sound of my heart monitor alarm going off down the hallway in the nurse's station and watching nurses sprint into my room. I remembered getting an infection, and how sick and feverish it made me.

I remembered being unable to sleep for nine straight days because my back hurt just as much as my chest did. The rib spreader shoved my chest and back muscles out of shape. I hurt no matter what position I was in. On my side, the two halves of my sternum scraped against one another, popping, cracking. I remembered hallucinating from lack of sleep.

Finally sleeping, and waking up feeling my sternum shift and crack as if hit by a sledgehammer. Feeling pain so severe I couldn't stop trembling.

I remembered being so fragile I couldn't use a remote control without crying from the pain. I couldn't move my arms. Couldn't hold a paperback book. Not for days, but for weeks afterward. I didn't laugh for two months. I couldn't play my cello without pain for a year. I couldn't have a hug without pain for two years.

It took two whole years to crawl my way toward recovery, and I'm still not the same. All of this I remembered, as the CT scanner hummed and the bed moved, and I held my breath while looking at the contraption holding the IV contrast dye.

The first time I waited to find out if I had a thymoma, I was scared of the unknown. The second time I waited, I knew exactly what to fear. Knowing how close I came to dying, how it felt when I first woke up from surgery, scared me even more. Going through that again was unimaginable. The memories played inside my mind like an out of control DVD and I didn't have the remote.

To my joy, my doctor called and said my chest CT was clear. There was no sign of a tumor. My cancer is considered cured! I danced and celebrated. Then I trembled even worse than before. Wow! How did I live through *that*? Once I knew I was past the physical suffering, I had to deal with the emotional whirlpool. The water was so deep and cold I thought I might drown.

I knew I needed help to get through it. At first, I felt silly asking for help. After all, it had been over six years. But, I've since learned emotions don't follow calendars. They freeze in time and stay just as powerful when the Later Box reopens.

From the whirlpool, I reached out to my friend, Hannah. She's a cancer survivor, too. Having lived through the whirlpool herself, Hannah just talked to me for hours, reassuring me that I was OK. Comparing notes with someone who took some of the same classes at The University of Catastrophe helped a lot. Finding a thymoma cancer patient support group helped as well.

Six years later, finally talking about what I'd been through let me start to heal. Accepting fear and trembling as part of letting go kept me from feeling like I was losing my sanity. Having cancer is scary, and even years later the fear and trembling are well deserved.

But, talking about it didn't stop the DVD from playing. The conveyer belt took me rapidly from diagnosis to surgery. It was all so fast and out of control, it didn't feel real. Apart from the scar on my chest, it felt like those memories didn't belong to me. It felt like something I'd seen on TV, not something I experienced personally. I felt trapped in a bizarre half memory.

Around my seventh anniversary, I composed a piece for solo cello called *4x3x2*, which was the size of my tumor in centimeters. In D minor, the dark grief I felt sang through my cello, and the memories became real to me.

Creating music helped me express what speech just couldn't say.

Then came the tears. Tears over the shock of it all. Crying because I had to go through such a horrible experience. Seven years later, I cried and grieved. Only then could I begin to put the shattered pieces back together.

In my journal, I wrote about all of the things I did to survive. How the thought of my daughter's face gave me the strength to keep going when dying was easier than surviving. The courage it took to get up from the hospital bed and walk five whole steps to a chair. I began to honor my victories one after another.

Once I started honoring my victories, something unexpected happened. My victories became an epilogue for the rotten memory DVD. So, instead of remembering with a sense of out of control doom, I honor what I did right when everything went wrong. Instead of trembling when I think about surgery and the fight to survive, I feel a swell of joy. I made it! Yay! It was horrible and traumatic, unfair and hard. But, I survived and that makes me victorious.

Since then, I've learned to film epilogues for many of my rotten memory DVD's, and not just the ones I have about thymoma. When my brain randomly selects a memory and pushes play, I watch it through. Then I remember to honor the right choices I made under terrible circumstances. Honoring what I did right brings me hope and strength. It gives me back the control Nightmare Creek washed away.

Surgery took power from me and left me broken. But, long before my body healed, I started taking my power back. A month later, I started planning my flower garden.

I knew I wanted all different narcissi. Pure yellow daffodils, and yellow with orange center narcissus. I wanted purple tulips and pink hyacinths. I planned where I would put each flower. Three months to the day after surgery, I planted bulbs in my garden. Digging in the dirt made my still healing bones ache. But, I worked and worked in my garden until I planted each bulb. Then I rested. In the spring, I sat on a bench surrounded by flowers.

Every spring when the flowers bloom I remember I survived. Sitting on the bench with my cello, while surrounded by flowers growing and stretching under the sky, I celebrate life. With music and laughter, I honor the struggle it took to return to the land of the living. The gift of life is precious to me and I treasure still being alive.

Right now, I'm losing what most women prize in our society. My hair is gone. My eyebrows are thin and strange looking. The face I see in the mirror doesn't look anything like super models in magazines. But, I've discovered living is beautiful. Bald and sitting in a powerchair, I am alive. I am alive to see autumn turning to winter. Outside my window, I'm watching the first flakes of snow twirl in spirals on the leaves and grass. Watching the snow, I am alive to wonder. I am alive to love my family and friends. There is life in me disease cannot touch. Though I live permanently up Nightmare Creek without a paddle, I'm living strong as a maple tree and beautiful as the dawn.

Bitter Creek

Myasthenia gravis is a progressive, incurable, potentially fatal, neuromuscular disease. That's what my doctor told me. That's what I read on a myriad of web pages. But, I refused to believe it. I could not have an incurable disease. That was not acceptable. I was going to be cured. Understand? Cured.

So, I researched with all of my intellect and searched for a cure. Someone, somewhere, had to have figured out a cure for MG. If no one found a cure, I was going to discover one myself.

I learned how the neurotransmitter acetylcholine travels from nerve cells to acetylcholine receptor sites on muscle cells, causing muscles to contract. Acetylcholine is synthesized and stored in vesicles in the motor nerve terminal. T-lymphocyte antibodies destroy acetylcholine receptors, causing myasthenia gravis. I learned T-lymphocytes are a type of white blood cell formed in the thymus gland. The thymus gland is a lymphoid and epithelial organ that consists of lymphoid and epithelial cells. I even learned the thymus gland is located in the anterior mediastinum, behind the manubrium.

I studied diligently and deciphered medical jargon until I came to a final devastating conclusion: myasthenia gravis is a progressive, incurable, potentially fatal, neuro-muscular disease.

That pissed me off!

Equally as upsetting, my research kept coming across the phrase, "People with MG live normal lives." Obviously, whoever wrote that never had severe MG. I wake up in the morning and before I push the covers off, I'm already aware my arm muscles don't work like they used to. I swing out of bed, and lean on the wall for support.

I stagger to the bathroom. Sit on the toilet. Some mornings I can't get off the toilet because my thigh muscles switched off. When that happens, I call my service dog Honey to help me off the toilet. Otherwise, I grab the sink and pull myself back up. Then I struggle to grip my pajama pants and fumble with my clothes. I lean on the sink for balance and wash my hands. Brush my teeth. Choke on the toothpaste. Use my fingers to clear my mouth. Yes, this is a normal life. On Saturn! Before I had MG, I lived a normal life on Earth. I vividly remember… everything.

I remember what it felt like to ride my bicycle in the early summer. Miles and miles flying past, getting bugs on my glasses, dirt on my shirt. I remember pushing my muscles until they burned as I climbed steep hills, and the sense of accomplishment when I finally made it to the top. Pausing a moment to catch my breath, I watched finches and sparrows in the trees.

I remember guzzling water from my water bottle, and pushing the cap shut with my teeth. I remember climbing back on my bike and flying downhill – feet balanced on the pedals, holding on for dear life, with the wind in my hair. I remember riding my bike. Now my bike is underwater, captured by Nightmare Creek. A rusty pedal sticks up above the water, reminding me of what I've lost.

I remember washing my hair. The smell of citrus shampoo as I ran my fingers through my long dark hair while listening to the crackle of bubbles in my ears. I remember rinsing and rinsing all of my wonderful thick hair. I poured conditioner in my hands. I remember how my fingers slid through the strands as I worked the conditioner into my hair and ran a brush through all of the tangles. I started at the tips and worked my way up.

I remember finding a snarl and the sharp pull on my scalp. I added conditioner to the knot, worked it through with my fingers until the brush glided though my hair. Then I watched my dark hair turn white from the conditioner. After rinsing my hair and finishing my shower, I remember putting my hair in a towel while I dried off.

Once I was dressed, I divided my hair into three parts. Twist the left plait. Twist the right plait tight against my scalp, then braid. Left over center. Right over center. Again, again, again. I remember braiding my hair. Now I reach up and touch my scalp. Prickly in some spots, utterly smooth in others. Some hair grows, some hair falls out. With every cycle of chemo, my hair grows slower and slower, less and less comes back. My lovely long hair is gone. I'm bald. I see photos of myself and cry. I miss my hair.

I remember riding my bike and caring for my hair. They were so simple, so ordinary and normal, I didn't even know they were treasures until they were gone. I remember having a normal life. But, I don't have a normal life anymore.

I did not sign up for MG! When I was a kid and people asked me what I wanted to be when I grew up, I sure as hell didn't say, "I wanna be a bald lady who uses a powerchair!" Up until my late 20's, the most serious illness I ever had was an ear infection. Sick meant the flu. It did not mean permanent, forever sick.

Remember how I said the sum total of my life experiences added up to exactly diddlysquat? It's true. Before MG, I could think my way out of any problem. Using the same brain that earned me a 4.0 G.P.A. in college, I tried to think my way out of MG, but it didn't work. No matter how much I studied and learned, I couldn't change the outcome. I have a life threatening, progressive, disabling, incurable, nightmare disease. At 27, my whole future fell into a blender and some cosmic finger hit purée!

Why?

Why me? I'm a good person. I'm faithful to my husband. I'm a good mom. I don't break laws. I've never been arrested. I don't cheat on my taxes. I vote. I donate money to charity. I'm a caring, giving, loving person. So, what did I do wrong to deserve this? Which god did I offend? Zeus? Apollo? Ra? I'm sorry, all right? Can I have my life back? It's not fair! It doesn't make any sense, and sometimes I feel so angry I don't know what to do.

As MG slowly stole my muscle strength, more than anything, I wanted to know why. Maybe if I knew why it wouldn't hurt so much. Maybe I could make sense out of it, and give it some kind of meaning. But, just like I can't think my way out of this mess, I can't understand why, either. It's the age old question: why do bad things happen to good people? I still don't know the answer. I just know the question tore me apart and flung me into Nightmare Creek's swiftest whitewater rapids. This is where Bitter Creek merges with Nightmare Creek. Enraged, cold and bitter, I didn't know if I would survive the razor sharp rocks.

Bitter Creek was the beginning of an inward journey, which was just as tough to survive as surgery. MG tore my life apart. I wanted my life back, but it was gone. Without my consent, I mutated into someone I didn't recognize in the mirror.

I never wanted to be this woman, the one who struggles to move from place to place. Intellect wasn't going to save me from drowning in rage. In fact, my intelligence made everything harder. I kept going in mental circles, trying to figure out why this disaster happened to me. The more I tried to understand why, the angrier I got.

Slowly, I realized there are a lot of things in this world that I don't understand. I don't understand why my microwave works. Don't try to tell me, because as soon as you say *magnetron* my eyes glaze over. All I know is I put food in the box, push the buttons and my cream of mushroom soup gets hot. If it doesn't get hot, I throw the microwave in the trash and buy a new one. I don't need to know why the microwave works to use it. And I don't need to know why I have MG to deal with it. Once I finally understood I was asking the wrong question, the whitewater rapids ended.

I don't need to know why me. That's an unsolvable equation. Pondering why bad things happen to good people is best left to philosophers and the clergy. In the end, why me is irrelevant.

The deeper question is, "Now that it is me, how am I going to manage?" Somehow I had to adapt. I had to accept the unacceptable. I had to put the shattered pieces of my life into some kind of order that worked. Those changes had to come from within. I had to reach inside myself and find out who I was, and how to be the woman I didn't recognize in the mirror.

The Towel

While I was taking the University of Catastrophe class, *Everything You Never Wanted To Know About Myasthenia Gravis*, I learned about all of the symptoms: difficulty seeing, smiling, chewing, swallowing, speaking, moving, and rarely, breathing. Obviously, none of those things were going to happen to me. Until they did.

The first time I slurred my speech, I was stunned. I could feel what was wrong. My tongue pulled back in my mouth and wouldn't extend all the way to my teeth. No matter how hard I tried, I couldn't make my tongue work. I knew slurred speech was a symptom of MG, but never dreamed it would happen to me.

I took a Mestinon tablet, and half an hour later, I could talk again. I swear Mestinon works like spinach does for Popeye. All day, my muscles turn on and off like out of control light switches. Some days are better than others.

Still, when I slurred my speech for the first time, it felt like I fell down a flight of stairs and landed flat on my back. Turns out, life with a progressive disease often feels like falling down stairs.

Tumble, tumble! Bang! Ow! Dang-it! Whew! OK, I stopped falling. I'm all right. I can live with a cane. It's not so bad. As long as nothing else goes wrong, I'll be fine.

Just when I got used to a cane...

Tumble, tumble! Bang! Ow! Dang-it! Whew! OK, I stopped falling. I'm all right. I can live with a walker. It's not so bad. As long as nothing else goes wrong, I'll be fine.

Just when I got used to a walker...

Tumble, tumble! Bang! Ow! Dang-it! Whew! OK, I stopped falling. I'm all right. I can live with a wheelchair. It's not so bad. As long as nothing else goes wrong, I'll be fine.

Just when I got used to a wheelchair, I started slurring my speech. Frustrating? Yeah. I kept waiting for the progression to stop, for nothing else to go wrong. Every time my disease progressed, I shattered inside. Then I'd put myself back together, get used to my new limitations, only to shatter again when my disease progressed.

Well, that got depressing! I felt so frustrated it made me want to throw in the towel. I felt bitter and hopeless. I decided there had to be a better way of handling this mess. Maybe I should try having a positive attitude. People told me, "You gotta stay positive, Marie." Could a positive attitude help? I decided to give it a whirl.

Instead of focusing my attention on what I lost, I started paying more attention to what I could still do. This grateful attitude lifted my spirits and I pressed on like *The Little Engine That Could*. I chugged along, laughing at my body as I walked like a drunk duck in a hurricane. Determined not to let MG ruin my life, I focused on overcoming every obstacle. Once I had a positive attitude, I thought I had a handle on the situation.

Then my ability to chew and swallow faded. My diet gradually shrank to soft easy to swallow foods that didn't require much chewing. Bananas, puddings, cream soups, eggs and the like. Do I like eating eggs, cream soups, puddings and bananas? No. I like crunchy tacos. I like Caesar salads. I like beef jerky. I like juicy steaks. What I liked I couldn't eat anymore. Losing the ability to chew and swallow was a painful blow, and not just because of hunger.

You may not have given it much thought, but there is more to eating than just eliminating hunger. Around the world, people celebrate everything from births to funerals with food. What would a birthday be without cake? Mass without Holy Communion? Thanksgiving without turkey, stuffing, and gravy? Passover without lamb? Superbowl Sunday without spilling beer and salsa on your shirt?

Food is a huge part of our lives. We dedicate rooms in our homes to preparing food and eating it together. Even in our modern electronic age, newlyweds still receive pots and pans, silverware and china plates as gifts. Not being able to eat socially isolated me and that hurt more than hunger. There was nothing positive about losing the ability to chew and swallow. It was a devastating loss.

I remember going out to dinner to celebrate my dad's birthday. We went to a Chinese buffet. My favorite buffet. After I ate two bites of an egg roll, my mouth was done eating for the night. Stomach growling, I watched everyone eat plateful after plateful. There was nothing I could do but sit and watch. The suffering in my soul far outweighed the ache of hunger. I longed to connect with everyone at the table, but I couldn't do it. Conversation revolved around food.

"Wow, that General Tso's chicken is awesome."

"That stuff's hot! I'm still sweatin'."

"Me, too."

"I had some of that earlier. Too hot for me."

"Steve, you're such a wuss."

"Thanks, I love you, too. Hey, Dad? What's that? The stuff with the shrimp. Is it good?"

"It's pretty good. Here, try some, Steve."

All around me everyone enjoyed eating and one another's company. I sat in my wheelchair in silence, looking at the cold egg roll on my plate. I picked up the egg roll, tried to make my mouth move enough for one more bite. I failed. That night I had tears for dinner, and it wasn't the only time. Nothing made me feel more like a stranger in my own body than losing the ability to chew and swallow. It hurt. Being grateful for my family's company wasn't enough to hold back the pain.

I think it was during dinner with my family that I realized a positive attitude doesn't help much here in Nightmare Creek. It might look helpful from the shore, but here in the cold water, the only way to stay positive is to pretend. Allowing myself to have tears for dinner cleared the way for me. That night, I allowed myself to feel exactly what I was feeling without shame or apology. It felt like taking a deep breath of clean air to simply be real with myself.

The Journey

People often tell me to keep a positive attitude. I tried that. It was totally exhausting. No one can keep a positive attitude 24 hours a day, seven days a week. It's too much work. Worse, I ended up deluding myself. Being perpetually grateful forced me to lie to myself and deny how I really felt. Giving myself freedom to feel allows me to express myself. If I can express myself, I can be myself in any situation. Happy or sad, laughing or sobbing, it's all real and valid. When I was busy being positive about everything, I had to deny pain and pain is part of my life.

Sometimes my life is awesome. Like tonight when I was playing my cello and I found high D without missing. Not just once accidentally, but over and over. Didn't even slide up to it. Nope, I shifted up an octave and nailed that sucker to the wall. If you're not a cellist, that probably doesn't sound exciting, but trust me, for a cellist, that's like kicking a field goal from 52 yards. Here's the snap, the kick is up and it's... *good!* Third finger leaps on the fingerboard, hits the note and it's... *good!* I felt like slapping the universe a high five.

Then again, sometimes I feel like the universe slapped me and I'm left in tears. Both things happen to me, and you, and everyone else. That's life. Life flows up and down. Sometimes life turns us inside out. But, we can't quit and throw in the towel. Even when life hurts, and I know what it feels like when life hurts.

When I'm tempted to throw in the towel, I know it's time to use it instead. It's time to get a fluffy purple towel out of the linen closet and bring it into the bathroom. I turn on the faucet and fill the bathtub. While the bath is filling up, I light all of my favorite candles and turn off the lights. I get out my bath oil and add it to the running water. Soothing sweet pea fragrance fills the air. Maybe I'll treat myself to a mud mask facial. It's a whole lot easier now that I don't have hair! Ease my weary body into the tub and just relax. With a mud mask drying on my face, I settle myself inside.

I've gotten better at giving myself permission to rest. Permission to rest came side by side with the freedom to feel what I'm feeling instead of staying positive. I've learned to tune in to my body. Eat when I'm hungry. Rest when I'm tired. Reach out when I'm lonely. Instead of forcing myself to stay positive, I allow myself to feel upset and cry. After all, an upsetting thing is happening to me. It's OK for me to get upset sometimes and wrong to pretend I'm always happy. No matter how I feel, it's easier to be real.

Whenever I'm tempted to throw in the towel and give up, I treat myself gently, recognizing that my life isn't easy and struggling is OK. When life gets too hard, I stop and surround myself with things I love like fragrant candles and bubble bath. In the tub, I soak off the stress and frustration. Then I get out and dry myself off. Instead of throwing in the towel, I hang it up on the rack for next time. Cleansed and refreshed, I'm ready to face whatever comes my way.

Maybe Someday

When I tell people MG is incurable, and I'll be taking chemo in some form or another for the rest of my life, sometimes they pat me on the shoulder and say, "You don't know that. Maybe someday there will be a cure for MG."

Reading along, you may have thought that yourself. Maybe I'm wrong. After all, I don't have a crystal ball. There are new treatments for all sorts of diseases every day. Maybe someday there will be a cure for myasthenia gravis.

Maybe someday.

For years I wrestled with maybe someday. Kicking, screaming, and punching, I fought to get my life back from this nightmare disease. I went to countless doctor's appointments hoping it was maybe someday. But, it wasn't. Searching the internet, reading clinical trials, I hunted for a cure on the horizon. Weeks of seeking become months, and months turned into years. Still no sign of a cure. Hoping for a cure that never came sank me into depression.

One of Nightmare Creek's most dangerous passages is a narrow canyon. There are tall cliffs on either side and the water moves slowly here. There is no danger from rapids smashing you into rocks. The danger is getting stuck in the muck at the bottom of the creek bed. No warning signs let you know it's a trap.

But, it is a trap.

Fighting past exhaustion, you kick and fight to free yourself from the mud. You look up at the tall cliffs and remember the life you knew before The University of Catastrophe changed your life. What you want more than anything is high and out of reach. Here, hopelessly mired in muck, is where you wait to be rescued... maybe someday.

When people tell me, "Maybe someday there will be a cure," I know they mean well. They're trying to offer me hope, but it doesn't help at all. Maybe someday leaves me feeling hollow inside. Do you know why?

Imagine it's the hottest day of the year. A big storm blew through and your electricity has been out for days. Since the storm there hasn't been a hint of a breeze. You're sweaty and thirsty. Now, imagine someone hands you an empty glass and says, "Maybe someday there will be water in here."

That's not what you need. When you're hot and thirsty, you need water. You can't wait for maybe someday. Neither can I. Maybe someday satisfies my soul like an empty glass quenches thirst.

No matter how hard I struggled to get my life back, the MG thief was bigger and stronger than me. I might as well try pushing over a brick wall with my fists. Nothing I can do will give me back my old life. Even if a cure came tomorrow, my old life would still be gone.

Physically, I'd be able to run and ride my bike, swim and play. But, the memories would still be with me.

Sad truth is, my life before MG is gone. MG changed my body forever. However, I am not just a broken body. I'm me, and I'm OK.

The only way I could free myself from the muck at the bottom of Nightmare Creek was to quit struggling. I had to stop fighting a war I couldn't win and surrender to reality. Myasthenia gravis is a progressive, incurable, potentially fatal, neuromuscular disease. Over MG there can be no victory for me. Maybe someday there will be a cure, but I cannot put my life on hold until maybe someday. All I have is now. Right now, I can choose to keep my fists balled in frustrated rage. Or, I can open my hands and reach up toward the sunrise.

It took years to fully unclench my hands and reach up. I took a shortcut when I tried the positive attitude approach. It didn't work. There aren't any shortcuts in Nightmare Creek, but there are plenty of traps. It's easy to get stuck faking a positive attitude, or trapped in bitter despair. Once I freed myself from the muck, I left behind the woman I was, and embraced myself as I am now.

When I wake up in the morning, I no longer expect to jump out of bed. I don't rage when I teeter. I struggle to move and that's all right with me, now. Although I'd welcome a cure, I don't need a cure to be well.

Being well has more to do with what's going on inside my soul, than how my body works. I didn't know that before I got sick, but I do now. It's possible to be seriously ill and doing well at the same time. I think I really understood that when I got my purple power wheelchair.

After spending the summer of 2004 confined to a ten step radius from the nearest chair, getting my powerchair freed me physically. It did wonders for me emotionally and spiritually as well. No longer was I trapped in a body that didn't move. I could move with just the touch of a joystick. I wasn't confined anymore. I was free.

One of my first powerchair adventures retraced the route I used to ride on my bike. I went west on the Illinois Prairie Path, over the North-South Tollway, and down to the metal bridge over the DuPage River. Watching the river flow under the bridge, I realized I hadn't been that far away from home alone in years. The freedom I felt was indescribable.

No, I wasn't on my bike with the wind in my hair. But, I was able to get to my favorite bridge and able to watch the water dance and sparkle over the rocks. It was then I realized legs are overrated. It's moving that matters. Finally moving easily for the first time in years filled me with celebration. On that bridge alone, I spun in happy powerchair circles. I was overcome with joy simply because I could move.

Powerchair motors whirring, I continued on my way west along the trail. Seeing the sky over me and trees changing colors, I knew I was OK. My body might have changed, but the core of me – what makes me who I am – was just fine.

Light crept back into my life. I finally understood I could still be myself in this body, completely me and not a shadow of my former self. My former self is gone. I don't need her back. I don't spend my life grieving her passing. My hands are open and the fists are gone.

Working through MG weakness in my arms and hands, I play my cello from my heart. My cello's voice and

I laugh, sing, and dance. I can celebrate victories, or sing of dark times, getting tears on my cello. Then I can dry my tears with a new song, singing about the wonder of it all.

Knowing what I've already been through, I look forward to what's up ahead. If it hurts, I'll handle it. I know how to grieve and cry. I also know how to rebuild after my life shatters. If what comes next is fun, I'll enjoy it and celebrate with all I am. I welcome life, with all its ups and downs.

Seasons change and so do I. I've learned to bend and reach instead of breaking into pieces with every change in the wind. No longer a shattered mess, I've rebuilt my life wide enough to make room for MG. I've learned to be completely me – awake and alive, embracing life as it comes.

If maybe someday there is a cure for MG, I'll receive it with joy. If maybe someday never comes, that won't wreck my life. I'm alive and whole. With my hands open, I'm reaching toward the sky. If you can't understand why, maybe someday you will.

Monday

Tomorrow is Monday. Tomorrow is chemo day. I've been through so many cycles of chemotherapy I know exactly what to expect. First I'll sign in at the desk and pay my insurance co-pay. Then a technician will greet me. I'll get weighed and sigh softly at the weight I've put on. Steroids and weight gain go together like wine and cheese. Then I'll sit down in the blood test chair and get a blood test. I don't like getting my fingers stuck, so I'll try and pretend I'm brave. Except, I'm not brave. I'm a needle fearing coward and I'll wince when the little needle pokes my finger. While the technician squeezes my finger, I'll watch my blood drip in a little plastic tube.

Then I will wait for my blood test results – white cell count, red cell count, platelet count and other blood counts that make sense to my doctor and baffle me. Assuming they're all in range, I'll meet with my oncologist in a little exam room. We'll talk about how things are going. Then it's treatment time.

I'll leave the little room and go down a twisting hallway heading toward the treatment room. Ever wonder why doctor's offices have twisting hallways? It's so pa-tients won't escape.

In the treatment room, I'll pick a recliner. Hope-fully, the one by the fish tank will be empty. I'll watch the tinfoil barbs swim. Then I'll look around at the other re-cliners. Sometimes another patient will want to chat. Or maybe I'll just smile at people. Then I will get out my headphones and portable DVD player.

My chemotherapy nurse will come over and smile at me. We'll talk a bit. I'll try to pretend there's a new magic chemotherapy delivery system that doesn't involve needles. Meanwhile, my nurse will clean off my skin over my port-a-cath. Then she'll stick the needle in my port. Ow! Did I mention I'm a coward? It's true. I try to pretend I'm not an oversized seven-year-old. Except, sometimes I am an oversized seven-year-old! I hate needles.

Too scared to move, I'll hold still, looking away from my blood that's running into the IV tube. Then I'll glance over, see a small pool of blood on a greenish piece of waterproof paper. Ew! Why did I look?

My nurse will flush the IV line in my port. She'll tape the IV line in a loop over my port, then connect my IV line to a big bag of saline and a little bag of steroids. After that my nurse will inject anti-nausea medicine into the sa-line bag. Then she will turn on a blue pump and I'll watch the IV drip for a second.

After that, I'll turn on my DVD player and start watching *Star Wars*. Movies keep me from frantically chanting, "There is a needle in my chest! There is a needle in my chest!"

While all I'm getting is anti-nausea medicine and steroids through the IV, I'll feel fine. Then for some inexplicable reason, a nurse will show up with clear chemotherapy in two huge syringes. The first time I saw the syringes, I thought she was gonna stick me with the harpoons and I just about leapt off the recliner. Now I know all that Agent Orange is going in my IV bag. I also know I'm gonna feel like crap 20 minutes later.

The first wave of nausea always comes on subtly. Do I feel sick? Nah, that's my imagination. Keep watching the movie. Then I'll start to feel really lousy. The nurse will bring me an Ativan pill. I'll let it dissolve under my tongue. Ten minutes later the nausea will fade, and so will my mind.

I don't clearly remember what happens after that. I know I finish treatment and my husband drives me home. I know I lie down on the couch in the den. But, I have very little memory of what goes on between Monday afternoon's treatment, and Friday morning when I come out of the fog. It's all a bit hazy because of my anti-nausea medicines. I always sleep a lot. I take medication every six hours. My mouth tastes horrible and no amount of brushing or rinsing removes it.

Between Monday and Friday during chemo week, I'm awake for two hours, asleep for four. Wake up, eat three crackers and a little chicken. Awake for one hour, asleep for five. I have no concept of what day it is. I feel startled on Friday morning when I come out of the chemo cave.

I feel a little better on Friday, but I don't have much of an appetite. If I eat too much, I'll puke. I found that out the hard way! The Saturdays after chemo I eat constantly. I haven't eaten much more than a snack in days. Ravenous doesn't describe how I feel Saturday. The metallic taste in my mouth fades over the weekend.

By the following Monday, I feel great. Well, great for me, anyway. My muscles work. I'm strong enough to play my cello and enjoy my life. I'm feeling healthier than I have in years. That week goes by. Another week. By Saturday, I'm having trouble moving around. Sunday I'll struggle to chew and swallow. And on Monday morning, it will be chemo day again.

One week feeling terrible, two weeks feeling better. I've done this so often, it's become as routine as putting on socks and that stuns me. How in the world can chemotherapy become a routine? I have a chemotherapy appointment tomorrow and I'm not dreading it, worried about it, or even upset. Right now, I'm upset because I'm *not* upset.

The medical conveyer belt keeps hauling me forward. I can rage, but it still drags me toward Monday. I can panic, but the sun rises Monday morning with my consent or without it. Perhaps blending chemotherapy appointments into my routine makes riding the conveyer belt easier. Perhaps it's my mind's way of going with the flow, because if I really stopped and thought about it, I'd be like George Jetson, yelling, "Jane! Get me off this crazy thing!"

Or perhaps I've added chemotherapy into my life like a toll plaza on life's highway. I pay the chemotherapy toll and get to continue on my way. When I'm traveling, I don't think about toll plazas. I think about the song on my iPod, the view of placid cows out the window, the rain clouds up ahead. Toll plazas are just a small part of the journey. Tomorrow, I'll go to my appointment, pay my toll and then continue on my life's journey. The tolls are worth it, because life is worth it.

Sandcastles

The treatment room where I get my chemo is a comfortable place. There are recliners to sit on, TVs to watch, and even a fish tank with the largest tinfoil barbs I've ever seen swimming around peacefully. It's the only place I go where bald women are the norm. Settled in my recliner, I sometimes talk to other women while we get our chemo. We lament lost eyebrows, talk about that weird eyelash itch, and of course exchange ideas on where to get new hats.

Invariably, the question, "So, what kinda cancer do you have?" comes up. Explaining that I don't have cancer usually results in either puzzled or horrified looks.

In a way, I envy the people who are fighting cancer. Many of them will endure a limited number of treatments and walk away free from disease. Watching them, I wish I had cancer instead of MG and I could walk away free from disease, too.

Then again, there are people who get chemo at the same time as me who are clearly at the end of their lives.

Chemo is buying time, only there is precious little time left. Me? I'm living somewhere in between.

No matter what doctors do, they can't cure me. Hopefully, I can keep going for years. I'm a fighter. I've made it ten years. I can make it ten more. Yet, I'm still aware I'm living inside a sandcastle at high tide. Through the sandcastle windows, I can see the waves. I watch them come and I can't do anything to stop them. I'd move to higher ground, but there isn't any.

Every day, the surf pounds the sandcastle. The ramparts fell years ago. The drawbridge collapsed last spring. The battlements came under assault in the summer. From the corner tower, I watched as sand slipped away and waves battered the guard house.

Progressive disease steals abilities slowly, so I can watch it happening. It feels like my MG progresses stepwise. Sometimes, I have severe exacerbations where I lose ground quickly. In 2004, I went from walking normally, to using a cane, a walker, and a wheelchair within four months. Then, for no apparent reason, the disease slowed down. I regained a little ground. But, I never gained back everything I lost.

It's like falling down ten stairs and climbing up four. When I'm falling, I wonder how I'm supposed to live without something, only to get that skill back. For a little while I'm holding my own. Then without warning, MG wakes back up and attacks me again. I fall down ten steps, and slowly climb up four.

What was an unthinkably terrible day five years ago is a good day now. Late at night, I sometimes wonder if an unthinkably terrible day now, will one day be a good day.

Knowing my body is eroding is the hardest thing in my life, harder than actually losing skills. I'm aware of what's happening to me, and not sure of what's up ahead. For me, aggressive MG is as relentless as the tide.

When I get treatment, I often wonder about the people in the recliners around me. How long have they been fighting? Is their disease beatable? Or are they like me, living inside sandcastles at high tide?

I think the battle to beat cancer takes a totally different mindset than living in a sandcastle. You must go to war against cancer. Screw up all your courage, all your strength, all your hope and fight back. Chemotherapy is a sharp sword. Every treatment slashes the cancer monster until it dies. Then there is a celebration, a victory dance of joy. And there should be! Surviving cancer is worth celebrating.

I've slowly realized, since my disease is incurable, there isn't going to be a celebration for me. Every day the disease tide rolls in, wave after wave, while I watch the sandcastle dissolve and pray the keep holds.

I find this shockingly cruel.

It's especially painful when I'm getting my 17th infusion and the person next to me is cheering, "This is my last chemo! I made it! Six whole cycles! I did it!"

I'm delighted for them. And jealous as hell. Nurses congratulate the person next to me. I watch and listen to the cheering, knowing they will never congratulate me. I'm fighting for my life, holding the chemo sword, but I can't kill the monster. No matter how hard I fight, the sandcastle will collapse with me inside it.

This is when I give myself permission to despair. If I didn't despair, I wouldn't be human. I'd be lying to myself and the world, pasting on a plastic smile, pretending to be happy when I'm not. Myasthenia gravis sucks. Getting sick at 27-years-old really sucks. For some unknown reason, I drew the short straw. So, I give myself full permission to rage, despair, cry, and feel sorry for myself. Whenever I need to meltdown, I meltdown. Then I take a deep breath and stand up again.

When the tears dry, and I quiet down inside, I remember chemotherapy isn't always a sharp sword. Sometimes, it's a sand pail and a shovel. Instead of stopping the disease tide, the medicine helps rebuild the crumbling sandcastle.

Now that the ramparts are gone, waves assault the keep. Chemotherapy dumps new sand at the base of the keep and packs it in hard, restoring what was lost. It fortifies the keep, strengthening every crack. Each cycle the sandcastle is reinforced. For now, the keep is holding and all I have is now.

The battle to live inside a sandcastle at high tide isn't about fighting off a monster, like fighting cancer. It's about fighting to maintain what I already have. I have a family and friends who love me dearly. I have my cello. I have a life that matters. What I have is worth fighting for, and so I fight to stay here in this sandcastle.

Here in my sandcastle, I refuse to live a half full life. I flatly refuse to surrender my laughter, joy, hope and love to the waves. These things I keep in the highest tower, farthest away from the disease tide. Here in my sandcastle, I quietly celebrate life itself.

Questions

As you can imagine, I have a lot of questions about my life. Most of them are about my health. Will I live to see a cure for myasthenia gravis? If a cure comes, will it work for me? How come I have such aggressive MG? With treatment, most people with MG live normal lives. How come I don't? Am I always going to be stuck taking Mestinon and drooling from the side effects, or will a new drug help? Will a new drug let me stop taking chemotherapy? I'd love to never take chemo again.

More importantly, will I always be able to play my cello? I don't think I could live without my cello. My shoulders are weak and playing is getting challenging. My MG symptoms push through all the medicines with no problem. I'm not in remission. Not even close. What if chemotherapy fails? What then? An experimental bone marrow transplant? I've lived through so much already. Can I survive that, too? How long will the sandcastle hold?

I don't have any answers, just questions. No one has any answers for me, either. These questions challenge

me every day. When I share my questions, people sometimes say, "Take it one day at a time."

Great advice, but I can't switch off future tense and
never think about tomorrow, next month, or next year. I
can't pretend tomorrow doesn't exist, and I can't live as if
tomorrow doesn't matter. It does matter! My future is
shrouded in a mist. Should I plan for retirement? Think
about long term care insurance? Should I assume I'll live a
normal lifespan? Or, is it more realistic to realize Nightmare Creek has a deadly waterfall and the current is
slowly pulling me toward it?

When I think about this, I realize quality of life is
more important to me than the number of years. If something interferes with my quality of life, I take it seriously.
Above all else, it's extremely important to protect my
spirit.

My body does what it does. Medications change my
thinking, erase parts of my memory, and play games with
my emotions. All that's left is my spirit. If something
wounds my spirit, I take action to correct it.

A real sandcastle is held together with wet sand.
The sun, the rain, the tide, or a jerk can all destroy it.
Doesn't take much to upset the balance and collapse a
sandcastle. It's the same for me. My spirit holds my life
together. When my spirit is wounded, my survival is
threatened because my spirit is my strength.

If a toxic relationship sucks the joy out of my life,
I'll sever the relationship to protect my spirit. If something
as minor as a TV show bothers my spirit, I'll change the
channel. I've learned to tune in to how my spirit is doing.
Tuning in is how I keep the questions from destroying me.

It would be so easy to give up under the weight of my unanswerable questions. I've been through so much, sometimes I wonder if I can keep going. Sometimes I wonder if giving up makes more sense than fighting.

Have I ever seriously considered eating a gun? Of course I have! Knowing I'm not going to get better is hard. It shakes my faith, my courage, and my hope. People have committed suicide over less. My two choices are progressive, incurable, disabling disease. Or suicide. Which is better?

I know what is better for me. Life is better. Because I choose life, people tell me I have a positive attitude, but that's not always true. I allow myself to be negative and depressed. I allow myself to question and grieve. I don't always have a positive attitude, just like I don't always have a negative attitude.

What I do have is a quiet understanding that everyone has a major at The University of Catastrophe, and MG is mine. I'd change it if I could, but I can't. As challenging as the classes are they don't overwhelm me, and neither do the questions. MG and the questions are a part of my life, but they don't control my life. I do.

Rising to the occasion is a choice I make. Sometimes, I make that choice by instinct. Survival is the most basic instinct we have. Sometimes, I make a conscious choice to keep going. No matter what happens, or how hard it is to endure, I choose life.

I choose life by giving myself freedom to feel whatever I'm feeling. Elated, devastated, overwhelmed. I've learned to recognize what I'm feeling and give it a name. I've learned shutting off my emotions shuts down my spirit. Expressing how I feel either though words in my journal, talking to a friend, or through my cello, allows me to be myself. It's why I'm still here dancing.

I believe in celebration and wonder. I believe in life before death. Today is the first day of spring. Right now I'm celebrating surviving a tough Chicago winter. I was so ill last year, I didn't know if I would live through this winter. Not only did I survive winter, I had a ball. I composed music, enjoyed evenings by the fire with my family, cooked hearty meals and could actually chew and swallow them. Winter is over and I made it. This spring I have much to celebrate and little to mourn.

Celebration is easy for me. I'm aware that life is unfair in my favor most of the time. It's completely unfair that I have a warm place to stay on a cold night. Too many people don't have anywhere to go. If life was fair, everyone would have a warm place to stay.

Yes, it is unfair that I'm sick. It's also unfair that too many people have no access to healthcare. If life was fair, everyone who needed medical care would receive it. Remembering that life is often unfair in my favor helps me keep a balanced perspective. My spirit thrives on balance. She doesn't like chaos.

I'm finding questions without answers cause inner chaos. If I push the questions away, refuse to acknowledge them, they twist around in my guts like an egg beater whipping meringue. That inner churning throws my spirit out of balance. Dwelling on the questions in my life drops me into an abyss of despair, and that too throws my spirit out of balance.

The Journey

The tiny place between shoving away the questions, and dwelling on them, is where I dance. It's not a very big space. It's just big enough to spin my powerchair in joyful circles under a blossoming maple tree.

Branches block the view of the sky, but don't shut it out entirely. When I look up, I can still see through the branches and find the sky. Even though I have questions, I still can see through the trouble in my life and find the joy.

Solder Lines
(for Kim)

There is a stained glass studio in our basement with bins full of colored glass panes, glass cutters, flux and solder. I love making stained glass, and seeing many pieces of broken glass gradually come together to form something new and beautiful. Whenever I see stained glass for the first time, I admire something most people overlook: the solder lines.

Solder is the glue that holds the pieces of colored glass together. When I look at stained glass, I admire the solder lines because they reveal the artist's vision. The more solder lines there are in a stained glass window, the more interesting it becomes. It's not the big intact glass pieces that make stained glass beautiful, but the broken pieces held together with solder. I'm finding this is true for people as well.

Just about every day, someone pats me on the back and says something about my cheerful attitude. I usually nod and smile, while holding back tears. When people commend me for my attitude, I often wonder if they assume I woke up one day, shrugged my shoulders and said, "I've got MG. Oh well. Wonder who won the game last night?" Because, I didn't. I shattered. After surviving the Bitter Creek rapids, I was more broken than before. The dream of getting my life back drowned in the rough water. I was left utterly alone. No one was coming to rescue me.

When I got sick, pieces of my life no longer fit. I had to stop using my bike, cross country skis, snorkel and fins. I traded them for a cane, a walker and a wheelchair. My old toys are still in the garage, collecting dust and memories. As my body changed, and I lost muscle strength, I grieved each loss.

Grief sucks. Whether I'm grieving the loss of someone I loved, or the loss of a skill, it hurts. But, I've discovered grief is as much a part of life as laughter. It is a gift to be able to grieve. Grieving was the first step toward letting go of what was, and making something new out of what remained. Grief is like the copper foil that surrounds all of my stained glass pieces.

It's not enough to wrap foil around a piece of glass and put it back on the pattern. Unless I solder the pieces together, light will never shine through the colored glass. It'll just lay flat on my bench, incomplete and broken. My absolute favorite part is soldering the pieces of glass together. While the soldering iron heats up, I paint flux on the copper foil joints between the pieces. Flux is a smelly oily acid that makes solder flow.

Just like it's not enough to wrap stained glass pieces in copper foil, it's not enough to grieve the losses. Grief leaves me feeling incomplete and broken until I paint the shattered pieces over with determination. I'm determined to keep going, keep living, keep being me, even though my body is falling apart.

Painting the shattered pieces with determination takes courage. It's not easy to keep going after all hell broke loose in your life. It's easier to drown in Bitter Creek, or get lost in grief. Determination coats the losses with attitude, but that's still not enough to rebuild a shattered life.

When making stained glass, it is possible to put so much flux on the glass the copper foil peels off. I've done it before, and said more than a few obscenities afterward! It's possible for me to be stubbornly determined not to let MG get in my way. I'll try doing something I used to do with ease, only to discover my body doesn't move like that anymore. Then I have to grieve all over again. Determination helps, but attitude isn't strong enough to hold me together.

The solder I use in my glass studio is a mixture of lead and tin. The solder that holds my broken life together is a mixture of medicine, acceptance, and self-control. Accepting the unacceptable is a way of life for me. It took years to accept the changes MG made to my body. Acceptance doesn't mean I like it, because I don't, trust me. Acceptance simply means not fighting anymore. I'm not struggling to do the impossible. I know I can't ride my bike anymore. I know my limitations and I accept them. Wishing things were different doesn't make my legs move. Because I've grieved my losses and decided not to let them wreck my life, now I can accept life as it is, not how I wish it was.

I cannot control what MG does to my muscles. How I react, I can control. I can choose to cry, or scream, or howl with laughter. Depending on how I feel, those reactions are all appropriate.

I've learned self-control is tied to self-respect. Self-control is not about plastering on a big ole happy smile when my heart is breaking. I respect myself enough to cry when I hurt, laugh when I'm happy, and express myself fully through words and art. No matter what uncontrollable things MG does to my body, I can control my responses to them. Acceptance and self-control help me solder the shattered pieces of my life back together.

When I make stained glass, solder flows along the copper foil. The molten lead and tin shine brilliant silver at first. The shiny metal is beautiful until it oxidizes and turns a dull gray. Flux boils from the heat of my soldering iron and little flux beads sizzle and smoke. Carefully and slowly, I melt solder over all of the copper foil lines until no traces of foil remain.

In my life, I think the fire that keeps my determination, acceptance and self-control flowing is curiosity. Doesn't matter how tough the challenges are, or how frustrating, I am curious about what's next. Curiosity pushes me forward like an explorer wandering a new uncharted island.

I remain curious about the future, curious about how I'll adapt to the next challenge life throws my way. Sometimes, I wonder if my curiosity is irrational, but I'm still curious. I'm curious about the next song hidden on my cello waiting for my bow to find it. I'm curious about places I've never been and foods I've never tried. I'm curious about what the future holds for my family and friends. Life is a never ending buffet for me and I'm curious about… well, everything! Curiosity leads to discovery, and discovery leads to wonder. I live in wonder all of the time. What's next for me? I have no idea, but I'm on the road to find out.

I've learned how to sort the pieces of my broken life, letting go of what I can't do anymore. I've grieved the losses and reshaped my life into something new. It took time and hard work, but it was worth it.

Life is a struggle and we all get broken along the way. Maybe you have a few solder lines on your soul. Perhaps you have many. But, the story of your life is in your solder lines, and the story of your life is a matchless work of art.

For a long time, I thought what made someone beautiful was on the outside – flawless skin, hair, body. Now I know what makes someone beautiful is within. Where you shattered and came back together new and whole, that's what makes you beautiful. It's what makes me beautiful. I've come to treasure my solder lines. They crisscross and twist around like intricate Celtic knot work. My solder lines keep me whole.

The scars on my body surgeries left behind are life tattoos and I treasure them, too. I've survived many things, shattered and come back together more resilient than ever. I'm a kaleidoscope, a mosaic, an ever changing work of art, alive with color. No longer broken, I'm whole and new. I wouldn't have it any other way.

The Rant

It's a Monday morning and that means only one thing: I wanna talk about football. Every Sunday afternoon during football season I'm on the couch, sucking down beer, and cheering for the Chicago Bears. Yesterday was no exception. Did you hear that loud shriek? Yes, that was me, shouting as the defense snatched the ball out of the air and ran across the field with it. Interception and a touchdown! Whoo hoo! And, yes, I spilled beer and salsa on my shirt in my excitement.

The Bears are my favorite team. I live in Chicagoland and I grew up watching the Bears with my dad. That doesn't mean I only watch the Bears. Nope. I watch the Chiefs, Cowboys, Steelers, Packers, Browns, Colts, Broncos. . . I love watching football.

Every Sunday afternoon, I'm on the couch calling penalties as the yellow flags fly on the field. "Did you see that? That's holding on Number 27. That'll be another five yard penalty." Either that, or I'm yelling at the screen for the coach to throw the red flag and challenge.

"What incomplete pass? Are you crazy? It was a catch! He took four steps!" Or, "That wasn't a touchdown!

He never had possession of the ball!" Sometimes, I yell loud enough for the coaches to hear me through the TV and the red flags sail on the field. Yes, I'm a big help, I know. I'm convinced the entire National Football League couldn't function without me yelling at my TV.

Every Sunday I groan when some poor running back gets squashed. Here's the snap, the hand off, and... ooh, he's gonna need some ice. The sports guys say something about lost yardage on that play. Yardage? More like mileage. Ouch! I love watching sacks, turnovers, and missed field goals. Sunday afternoons, I'm drinking beer, eating jalapeño poppers, and yelling at football on TV. Monday morning my throat feels like I ate a porcupine. Who cares? I love football.

So, how come no one ever asks me about football? On a Monday morning during football season, people ask, "How's chemo going?"

How's chemo going? Unless I'm in the treatment room, it's not going. The only time chemo is going is when I'm sitting in the treatment room. Drip, drip, drip. Other than that, it's not going. Thank God! I'm mid cycle, finally feeling well and chemo is buried in my mind's locker room where it belongs.

Chemo? What's that? Don't you really mean, "Didja see the game? How 'bout them Bears!" It's Monday morning. Time for Monday morning quarterbacking. Do I get asked a single question about football? No. Of course not.

"Hi Marie. How's chemo going?" I hear it so often, I'm starting to think Howzchemogoing is my last name.

Forcing myself to use the manners my mother taught me, I mumble, "It's going OK." I attempt to change the subject to something really important like the current AFC football stats, but it never works. Way too often, the next thing I hear is, "Ya know, my mother's, neighbor's, best friend's, cousin's, hairdresser is on chemo."

And I am supposed to do exactly what with this information? I never know what to make of it. My heart does the equivalent of a shrug. It's not that I don't care what happened to their mother's, neighbor's, best friend's, cousin's, hairdresser. I do care, because I care about anyone stuck taking *Chemotherapy and You* at The University of Catastrophe. That class thoroughly sucks. I care, but my question is, why do people feel compelled to tell me about it? Are they trying to connect with me?

If someone wants to connect with me, they should ask me about... *football*. Putting me in a box with other bald chemotherapy patients is not connecting with me. I don't belong in a box. I belong in a conversation discussing who is the best quarterback in the NFL. Anyone ever ask me about that? No. They ask me about chemo, or my wheelchair.

"My nephew's, teacher's, veterinarian's, uncle's, father-in-law is confined to a wheelchair, too."

Another attempt at connecting with me that flies out of bounds at the 45 yard line. Wheelchairs and chemo. Chemo and wheelchairs. The two most obvious – and least important – parts of my life get discussed way too much. Is my life all about medicine and adaptive equipment? I guess it must be. Apparently, people using wheelchairs aren't allowed to love football.

Ever notice *invalid* meaning sick, is spelled the same as *invalid* meaning inconsequent? I can use them both in a sentence, "Since Marie is an invalid, her feelings are invalid." Not true? It sure seems that way.

Strangers ask, "What's the matter with you? How come you're confined to a wheelchair?"

If the question comes from someone under the age of 12, I answer politely and honestly with an open heart. If the question comes from an adult, I get angry. What kind of greeting is that? Not, "Hi," or, "How ya doing?" But, "I'm a total stranger; would you discuss your medical condition with me, because I'm nosy?"

I'm not really sure how to answer that. On the one hand, MG is an extremely rare and damn interesting disease. I'd never heard of mya-whatever-ya-call-it before I won the lottery in reverse. On the other hand, in the grocery store I'm a lady – who happens to be seated on a chair with wheels on it – shopping for a good deal on barbecue sauce. I'm not a side show act, or a rolling one woman freak show. Why I use a wheelchair is my business.

I have never asked a stranger when she had her last pap smear. Never asked a stranger how his prostate is doing. I don't even ask if it's boxers or briefs. Why people get offended when I refuse to answer nosy questions is beyond me. If I was standing and shopping for barbecue sauce, would the same stranger ask about my mammogram results? Of course not! Duh, that would be rude. Just because my medical condition is visible doesn't make it any less private. Doesn't make the wheelchair question any less rude, either.

Believe it or not, it's not my duty to tell everyone I meet why I use a wheelchair. I am allowed to go shopping without a note from my doctor, just like everyone else.

When people ask me, "So, why are you confined to a wheelchair?"

I really want to answer, "Why do you wanna know? Do you wanna borrow it? It's gotta be hard to walk with your head so far up your butt!"

But, my mom taught me manners and then set them on default in my brain software. She didn't give me the login code, so I can't uninstall the program. For some odd reason, Mom programmed me to greet strangers with, "Hello."

When strangers ask rude questions about my wheelchair, instead of snapping at them, I politely answer, "Because my flying carpet is in the shop." Then I roll away laughing.

This stupidity doesn't only happen at the grocery store. Since I'm using a wheelchair, I'm obviously incapable of reading a menu and ordering at a restaurant. "What will she have?"

What about getting on a plane? Can I do that? Nope. "Does she have her boarding pass?"

The last time I checked, the proper form of address, when speaking directly to someone, was *you*! "What would *you* like for dinner?" Or, "Do *you* have *your* boarding pass?" I may slur my speech sometimes and sound like I'm drunk, but I'm sitting on my butt, not my brain.

You would think I'd be safe from foolishness while powerchair cruising on the Illinois Prairie Path. But, I'm not. Imagine this. I'm taking my service dog for a 10 mile trot. The sun is shining. Honey is panting and grinning up at me. I'm cruising along, having a great time.

Then out of nowhere, a man flying past me on his bike yells, "No speeding!"

Wow! What an original thing to say to someone using a powerchair. You're so funny, you should have your own show on TV.

"No speeding, now. Mind how fast you drive that thing."

I've noticed that no one – absolutely no one – ever says that to someone who is jogging or riding a bike. But my powerchair, cruising at a whopping 6.5 miles an hour, is such a threat to the world speed record I need to be warned. "No speeding!" What a jerk!

Just once I want someone to say, "Hi. Beautiful day for a run." That'd be a touchdown with an extra point for the Able Bodied team. After all, that's what I'm doing in my powerchair. I have heels on instead of track shoes, but I'm still taking my dog for a run.

"What a lovely dog!" That's a field goal for the AB's.

"Hi!" Good enough for an AB first down.

However, petting the on-duty service dog without asking? That's a five yard penalty.

And, "No speeding!" Personal foul. Illegal use of the mouth. That's a 15 yard penalty and a loss of down for the Able Bodied team. The AB's will have to punt. You blew it. Go sit on the bench!

Sometimes people see my powerchair and say, "Wow, you drive your chair really well."

How often have I heard that? With a straight face, I usually answer, "You walk really well, too." Sometimes, they get it. Sometimes it's batted down and they just give me a blank stare. I turn away before I laugh. I do that a lot in public. So many people are unaware of how silly they sound.

I've actually had strangers ask if I know so-and-so who is confined to a wheelchair. For the last time, your ex-husband's, boss's, priest's, sister Penelope is not someone I know because I use a wheelchair. Wheelchairs do not come with an email list or a phone book. There is no clandestine underground of wheelchair users secretly plotting a takeover of the world. I know that may come as a shock to some people. Obviously! Otherwise, I wouldn't hear it so often.

I'm sure these people mean well. But, their attempts at getting to know me push me away. Just once, I want to have a conversation with someone and never hear the words chemo or wheelchair. I wanna talk about the current standings in the NFC North. Is it too much to ask?

Enough. I gotta watch football highlights on ESPN and talk to myself about the Bears chances of winning next week. Maybe someone will ask me about football tomorrow. But, then again, they probably won't.

The Rant Explained

Whew! Glad I got that off my chest. *The Rant* began after I received an email on a Monday morning. The day before, The Chicago Bears pulled off a spectacular win and I was psyched. It's not every day you see your favorite team turn a muffed field goal attempt into an NFL record breaking, 108 yard run back for a touchdown. That was totally awesome!

The guy on the TV said, "The kick is up... No good... Wait! Bears ball! Bears ball!"

Steve and I screamed, "Go! Go! Go!" as Nathan Vasher flew down the field. "He's at the 30! The 20! 10! Touchdown!" I got so excited, I spilled my beer on the couch. Steve flung onion dip on his dog. That was great!

Monday morning, I was surfing the web, watching game highlights, when my e-mail beeped. I clicked open my new e-mail and it was from an acquaintance.

She asked me how chemo was going, asked about my wheelchair repair, and told me about her friend who took chemo. I sat there looking at the email in frustration. This person was attempting to connect with me. I understood that. But, instead of drawing closer, I felt repelled. I didn't understand why until I clicked open my word processor and started writing. *The Rant* exploded out of me, a literary mushroom cloud of frustration.

There I was, having a blast studying football stats, when suddenly I realized no one ever asks me, "How 'bout them Bears?" Even when I wear a Bears hat and a Bears sweatshirt, no one asks me if I saw the game. While reading the e-mail, I felt like I was nothing more than a crippled chemotherapy patient to this person, and that really pissed me off!

Most people have no idea what it's like to use a powerchair, or sit in a treatment room while chemotherapy is pumped into their body. I get that. I really do. The idea of getting a serious illness is enough to make most people break out in a cold sweat. Severe MG is the stuff of nightmares.

But, if all you see in me is a nightmare, you haven't seen me. Hence, *The Rant*.

Perhaps if I was born disabled I wouldn't feel so frustrated. Or more likely, I'd feel differently frustrated. I can't speak about growing up disabled, because I spent the first 27 years of my life able boded. So, instead of growing up with disability incorporated into my sense of self, I've had to blend it into my adult life.

Giving up my bike and other average things I did without thinking about them were painful losses, true. But, not as painful as realizing people treated me differently. Special. Disadvantaged. This I found startling. It challenged my intellect.

Was all the work I did to incorporate MG into my life an exercise in futility? After all, I could be what all the stereotypes tell me I am. I could be bitter and angry, rolling around with a chip on my shoulder. I could scowl at people. I could yank the door out of someone's hand when they were just being polite. I could give up, stay home, hide from the world and all the foolishness people direct my way. But, then I would give up being me.

Since I've worked so hard to strike a balance between illness and the rest of my life, it takes me up short when someone points out my differences. It's not that I'm unaware of them. How could I be unaware? MG just matters so little compared to the rest of my life.

I'm a football fan. I cook a kick butt pot of clam chowder. I like *Star Trek* and *Doctor Who*. My favorite movie is *The Lord of the Rings: The Return of the King*. I love to read. I really enjoyed the *Harry Potter* books. My family still teases me because I inhaled *Harry Potter and the Prisoner of Azkaban* in one night. Hey, it was a good story. I've inhaled good books since I was three.

Knowing there is so much more to my life than disability and illness, I feel confused when people ask me about chemo and wheelchairs, wheelchairs and chemo. Yes, I know I'm bald. And yes, I know my wheelchair is purple. I picked out electric purple because purple is my favorite color.

Now that we have that established, can you recommend a good book? A new recipe? Seen any good movies lately? Can you tell me where you got your new black pumps? They're adorable! I missed Monday night football because I had a gig. Who won?

Small talk is welcomed. I love to talk about normal things because I am normal. My body might move differently from yours, but that doesn't make me abnormal. Different, but not abnormal.

Sometimes when I try to start small talk with someone, the subject of my wheelchair ends up in the conversation. Admiring my chair, much like someone admires a pretty jacket, is one thing. Nosy questions are another. I feel set aside when that happens. Pushed into the "them" category. What I want able bodied people to know is, I'm not struggling bravely with my problems. Or being brave by doing the ordinary. I'm just... me.

So if you see me during football season, and you notice I'm wearing a Chicago Bears jersey, call out, "How 'bout them Bears!"

You'll get an earful from me, either recounting a spectacular sack, or cheering over a touchdown. Or if they lost, I'll grumble about a fumble and wonder if the Bears need to go shopping at Quarterbacks R Us! Sometimes, it's tough to be a Bears fan.

One thing you won't miss is the happy expression on my face. I'll be grinning ear to ear, because you'll have done what a lot of able bodied people fail to do: see me for who I am. Go ahead, ask me about football. You never know, I might invite you over to watch next week's game.

Oh yeah, and one other important thing: Go Bears!

Life Jackets
(For Chris)

It happens all of the time. Someone on the shoreline sees me floating along up Nightmare Creek and wants to help. They call to me, holding an orange life jacket in their hands. Or at least, it looks like a life jacket. It's the right size and color. Only problem is it's filled with rocks. Without bothering to ask my consent, they force the fake life jacket around my neck and buckle it on. The second they strap it on me, I sink.

Meanwhile, the person who gave me the phony life jacket leaves, probably thinking, "Wow! I'm so glad I could help."

It never occurs to anyone their suggestion made me sink to the bottom of Nightmare Creek. They meant to be helpful, but their life jacket made it worse.

There are all kinds of fake life jackets people fling my way. They're based on stereotypes, myths, and just plain ignorance. Like this one, *"I know how you feel."*

Really? You mean you've lost your sight, gotten it back, gone through a sternotomy, watched your body fall apart, and taken chemo, too? Wow, we're twins!

Wait. No, we're not.

I usually hear, *"I know how you feel,"* when I'm feeling down and someone is trying to console me. It looked like a life jacket, but wasn't because the only person who knows how I feel is me. Unless you've attended some of the same classes at The University of Catastrophe, you can't begin to imagine how I feel. You can be compassionate and concerned, but you can't know how I feel. Just like I can't know how anyone else feels.

When I'm worried about my future, I sometimes hear, *"No one knows how long they're going to live. I could get hit by a train tomorrow."*

OK, this phony life jacket is filled with rocks, ball bearings, and wet cement. There is a vast difference between wondering about getting hit by a train, and being tied to the tracks with a train coming toward you.

For me, MG has been life threatening. It still weakens my breathing muscles. I choke on food several times a week and I don't have a proper gag reflex. My immune system is weakened and I could get a life threatening infection without warning. Next time I get a fever of 100.5, I have to go to the emergency room. Again.

I live on the tracks, watching a train coming toward me. I'm grateful that chemo made the train slow down. The train might have stopped moving, or maybe it's going backwards! I can't judge its speed. But, I'm still living on the tracks, and I can still see the train.

Telling me, *"I could get hit by a train tomorrow,"* cheapens my struggle. The people who say it are, again, trying to comfort me. I understand. Only, it has the opposite effect and leaves me feeling lonely inside.

I do not ask that you enter into my struggle, only that you respect its challenges. My reality is, the light at the end of the tunnel is the headlight of an oncoming train. All I can do is live my life in the path of a train, playing my cello on the tracks, and enjoying the time I have. I do my best to ignore the train whistle behind my back. It's loud sometimes. It is not an easy thing to ignore.

The worst thing I could imagine happening is someone I love getting hit by a train tomorrow. It doesn't console. It only frightens me.

Those are some of the more upsetting phony life jackets. But, there are others, more irritating than painful. Such as, *"You must have been a really terrible person in a past life to have to work off so much bad karma."*

Yes, some people actually say things like that to me. Yes, some people are jerks! I've known that for a long time.

"Have you tried prayer?"

That's a tough question to answer considering the number of deities people worship. If you're asking if I've sacrificed 100 oxen to Zeus in the past week, the answer is no.

"If you had enough faith, you could walk."

Know what? This makes me want to slowly roll my 300 pound powerchair over someone's foot. Crush every bone and say, "If you had enough faith, that wouldn't have hurt."

There is nothing wrong with faith. Faith can give people courage when nothing else can. Please don't get me wrong, I have nothing against God. It's just some of God's followers worry me. Especially when they say, *"God never gives you more than you can handle."*

Did you remember to send enough box tops to get your decoder ring? OK, get out your new ring so we can decode, *"God never gives you more than you can handle."* That's right! What they're really saying is, *"Better you than me!"*

Why do strangers see my wheelchair and then talk to me about religion? I've wondered about that for years. Perhaps it's to comfort themselves. Since they're praying to the right deity, reading the right holy book, going to the right religious services, and doing all of the right things, this horrible disaster won't happen to them. Therefore, I must have done something wrong to deserve this, either in this life, or a past life.

Maybe they don't realize their comments are fake life jackets. Maybe they think they're being helpful. But, being dumped overboard into Nightmare Creek challenges everyone's faith – their faith in God and their faith in themselves. Knowing I'm not going to get out of Nightmare Creek until I drown? Let's just say this doesn't make me feel like dancing for joy.

When people talk to me about religion, it fills me with questions that I can't answer. Questions lead me away from my hard won peace. When I hear, *"God never gives you more than you can handle,"* I don't feel comforted. I boil with rage.

Every time I hear, *"God never gives you more than you can handle,"* I end up having a screaming, crying, hysterical meltdown, because I can't handle this. It's too much. It's too cruel. I don't even know why it's happening to me. If God loves me, than why…

See? It stinks! And that's not the only thing that stinks. I can't tell you how many times I've been asked, *"Have you seen Dr. Quack? You're probably allergic to something like milk. Dr. Quack can help you find out what allergies you have so you can get better."*

Does Dr. Quack have any published data in *JAMA* regarding myasthenia gravis and milk? Get me a copy. I'd really enjoy reading it to my neurologist.

"Have you tried a coffee enema?"

No. I prefer my coffee orally for some odd reason. One cream, no sugar, please.

"Have you tried vitamins?"

Vitamins? Really? Why would I subject myself to chemotherapy when vitamins are the answer? Wait here while I ask my oncologist if I can switch to high doses of vitamin E.

"If you take these herbs, your immune system will go back to normal."

You're right. According to the front of the bottle, these herbs are incredible. I can't wait to try…

Oh, wait. The back of the bottle says, "These statements have not been evaluated by the Food and Drug Administration. Not intended to diagnose, prescribe for, treat, or claim to prevent, mitigate, or cure any diseases."

Hmm. Should I take your mystery herbs? Or should I listen to my doctors and keep doing what I'm doing?

"You must have internalized a lot of anger to make your cells attack your own tissues."

Warning! Warning! Danger! The more you speak, the more anger I'm internalizing. You might want to stop yapping before my fist releases my anger into your jaw!

"You should exercise more. Then your muscles will get stronger.

Let's review. If I use a muscle, it gets weaker. If I rest a muscle, it gets stronger. Exercise is the last thing I need. Rule number one with MG is energy conservation. Do you really want me to violate rule number one?

"Do you have an acupuncturist?"

As a matter of fact I do. But, I'm not interested in trading her in for a tarot card reader, astrologer, or a shoe-shine boy.

"Are you eating low carb? You should."

Low carb. OK. Bacon and eggs, hold the toast. Got it.

"Don't eat eggs. They're full of cholesterol."

OK, bacon. No eggs. I'm on it. Wait while I scrape these scrambled eggs in the dog's bowl. Here you go, Honey. Enjoy.

"Don't eat bacon. It's full of chemicals."

Scrape the bacon in the dog's bowl with the eggs and… Oh look, Honey is doing a happy dance. So much for breakfast. My dog eats better than I do. I'm hungry. What do I eat now?

"Are you eating enough whole wheat bread?"

No, I'm eating low carb.

"Don't eat low carb! You need a low fat diet."

I do? OK, I'll eat fish.

"No, don't eat fish! It's full of mercury."

Enough! I give up. My husband Steve always says, "If eating it makes you feel good, it's health food."

I'm with him. Hang on, let me get the cork off my Shiraz and…. Thunk! Glug, glug, glug. Fumble, fumble with a chocolate wrapper. Ah, now this is my idea of health food.

The life jackets filled with rocks always come my way from people who mean well. They see me up Nightmare Creek and want to help. The problem is, people don't always offer what would help me float.

How about instead of asking if I'm praying, just tell me, "I'll pray for you." I can use all the prayers I can get.

Since I have trouble moving around, shopping is tough for me. How about calling me on the phone and saying, "I'm on my way to the grocery store. Do you need me to get anything for you?"

If you go shopping for me please don't tell me what I should eat. Just offer to get the foods I enjoy eating. Red wine and chocolate will be on the list. That's automatic. Our neighbors Jeff and Julie have helped us out with groceries several times and I'm grateful.

Sometimes, I don't have the energy to make dinner. I can't count how many casseroles all of my neighbors have brought my family. It makes floating up Nightmare Creek easier when the entire neighborhood shows me they care.

Even friends who live far away find ways to cheer me up. My friend Nada just sent me a mini-marshmallow shooter. Perfect! I had fun shooting marshmallows for hours. I'm easily amused. If it made you smile or laugh, chances are it'll do the same for me.

When I started chemo, one of the best consolation presents I got was a gift card to a video store from my neighbor Peter. I bring a portable DVD player to the treatment room. I sit in a recliner for several hours, so a new movie is just perfect. I watched *Star Trek IX: Insurrection* last time. Very cool for an ultra space nerd like me!

Groceries, casseroles, marshmallow shooters, gift cards, these things are real life jackets, things that help me float. I would have drowned long ago without them.

When people we care about are up Nightmare Creek, it's hard to stand on the shore and watch. It's tempting to throw a life jacket filled with rocks, but I'm encouraging you not to toss one. Just take it from someone permanently up Nightmare Creek, platitudes don't help, but actions do.

If you know someone who is going through a tough time, I encourage you to toss a real life jacket. Offer to mow the lawn. Or do some of their laundry. Or baby-sit their kids. Maybe you could go grocery shopping for them. Make a casserole. Buy flowers. Or even mail a silly greeting card with a terrible pun inside. All of these things have helped me over the years, and they'll help someone else, too.

One of the best real life jackets is just quietly listening. I treasure the people in my life who really listen to me. I can rage to them. Or cry. Ask questions I know they can't answer, just to get them off my chest. Their stillness and acceptance help me find my own stillness and acceptance. I couldn't float without them.

Rock filled life jackets come my way under the assumption I'm not happy splashing around Nightmare

Creek. But, I am content. This is my home. I've found what works for me, and what doesn't. I'm already doing the right things, in the right way, to take care of myself. If I wasn't, I'd be dead.

So, instead of tossing out life jackets full of rocks, just talk to me about what everyone else talks about. Feel free to talk to me about thunderstorms and how your dog hid under your bed. I'll tell you about the time my husband's weimaraner got so scared during a storm, April cowered in the bathtub for three hours. Poor thing!

We can talk about our pets and shoe shopping, football and the news. Talk to me about life, and I'll give you life back. But unless I'm riding beside you in a boat, please do me a favor and leave the life jackets behind.

Hide or Seek

O ver 100 years ago, popular child rearing advice said, "Children should be seen and not heard."

When you have a disability, some people seem to think you should be neither seen or heard. They treat you like a dented can on a store shelf, something to be passed over and avoided.

Society has some strange hang-ups about wheelchairs. People say someone is confined to a wheelchair. Or wheelchair bound. But, a wheelchair is nothing but a tool that I use. It's just a piece of adaptive equipment that helps me function and enhances my quality of life. Adaptive equipment is more common than you realize. You might be using it right now.

Glasses and contact lenses are adaptive equipment. They are tools to help us function and they enhance our quality of life. Glasses are for eyes. Wheelchairs are for legs. That's the only difference between them. Except, no one ever talks down to you just because you're wearing glasses.

Imagine for a moment, what it would be like if you were in the grocery store shopping while wearing glasses, and a total stranger walked right up to you and said, "Oh, are you here all by yourself? Just look at you being so independent! I just think you people who have to wear glasses are so brave. You know, I have been watching you shop and I just had to come over here and tell you that you are such an inspiration to me, and I hope you have a wonderful day."

Wow! If that actually happened to you in the grocery store, just because you were wearing glasses, I bet you'd be thinking, "Huh, psychiatrist in a can. Now where did I see that? That's right! It's in aisle nine, right between the nuts and the fruitcakes. Wait here, because I'm gonna get you some."

OK, that condescending attitude toward a pair of glasses is obviously ridiculous. However, that same condescending attitude toward a wheelchair is commonplace. Everytime I have to deal with it, it makes me want to hide.

Want to know a secret? I hate being called, "Inspiring." Inspiring is a label people stuck on me that puts me in a box. It's a box full of stereotypes and assumptions that turn me into a caricature, instead of allowing me to be the whole person I really am.

The word inspiring comes from the Latin root word *inspirare*, meaning to give life, to give breath, to give spirit. When you inspire someone, you are giving of your spirit.

When I play my cello for people, that's a giving of my spirit. This book is a giving of the best of my spirit. I'm honored for every opportunity I have to give from my spirit. However, sitting in a wheelchair in a grocery store, we call that... uh, shopping. Shopping isn't an inspiring thing to do. It's about as ordinary as you can get.

Know what? Shopping while seated is slightly different than shopping while standing. Just like shopping while wearing glasses is slightly different than shopping while not wearing glasses.

But, when people receive someone with a disability, doing the ordinary – grocery shopping in a wheelchair, riding a bus while blind, signing to a friend in the mall – as if what they were doing was extraordinary and inspiring, it feels like that person just took spirit away. I call that dignity theft. Dignity theft is treating me as the sick person you know.

It's impossible to have a relationship with anyone when I'm just the sick person they know. The only thing we talk about are my illness and treatment. Never how their kid is doing in soccer, or how my daughter is doing in school. "How are you feeling, Marie?"

Annoyed. I find talking to you very boring. I would much rather talk about your beautiful begonias. But, I'm just the sick person you know, so all conversations must revolve around my illness. That's the rules.

I would far rather be a person you know. Then we can share life. My friends understand this. We talk about everything from pet turtles and cats, to scuba diving and seeing the coral. We talk about flower gardens and places we've been. We talk about their work and mine. We cheer each others victories and dry one another's tears.

My friends don't hesitate to tell me, "I've got a tummy ache." Or, "My allergies are kicking my butt." Or even call me on the phone and whine about having another cold. They know I'll care. They know they can count on me to cheer them on when things get rough. They know their stories will crack me up, or I'll have a story to crack them up. We enjoy one another's company and love each other dearly. My illness is in the background where it belongs, because we know each other.

I want to be known. Not invisible. I want people to seek me out instead of seeing only what's "wrong" with me. So much more is right with me than wrong.

Weaving Part I

(In memory of my Mom, the weaver & musician)

After I finished raging, stopped clenching my fists and opened up my hands, I had to figure out where MG fit in my life. Is it the center of my life? After all, it looks like the center.

It took a long time to realize neither MG or treatment are at the center of my life, because I am not a disease. I'm me. I'm living, breathing and growing. I'm not just existing, trapped inside a body that doesn't work. I've blended my disease into my life like stirring lemon into tea. It flavors my life with a bitter sting, but I'm not bitter.

My studies at The University of Catastrophe taught me this: trouble happens to everyone. Right now you are either currently enrolled, about to be enrolled, or a graduate of The University of Catastrophe. Everyone is born with a full scholarship.

I majored in aggressive myasthenia gravis, with a minor in thymoma cancer. I didn't pick my course of study at The University of Catastrophe. No one does. Life is not fair, but that doesn't mean it isn't good. My life is very good.

There is so much more to my life than MG. I'm a wife. A mom. A musician. A composer. A writer. A daughter, a sister, and a friend. I'm a stained glass artist. Did you know I train dogs? I love to cook. I fix computers. I play video games with my daughter. I give. I receive. I live. I laugh. These things are at the center of my life, the reasons I wake up in the morning and smile at the day. My problems are in the background, the dark backdrop on the tapestry of my life. MG is woven into my life and doesn't overshadow it.

The anger I felt, the bitter rage and pain, were the needle and thread stitching MG into my life – opening my life wider, cutting things away, stitching in something new. Colors appear brighter against a dark background, and my life is full of bright colors. I don't live despite disease. I don't live with disease. I just live. MG is a part of my life, and so is my smile.

On this journey, I learned to really feel. Joy and pain. Rage and stillness. I've learned to be true to myself. I'm free to panic, despair, grieve and rise above. When life knocks me down, I'm free to take as long as I need to unclench my fists and get up again. Life isn't a race. The time it took to solder my life back together was time well spent.

Now that my hands are open, I'm able to receive all the gifts life has to offer me. Sunlight dancing on the water. Music well played. A warm fire in our fireplace on a freezing Chicago night. I've learned to find joy in the simplest treasures. Talking with a friend. Evelyn and Steve goofing off in the kitchen. The quiet knowledge that I am dearly loved. These are the things that keep me going, the riches illness cannot take away.

The Journey

There is a light in my life nothing can dim. It's powered by my memories. Every time I could have quit, but didn't. Every time I could have lost hope, but didn't. Those memories are my fire. The knowledge I've gained on this journey lights my way. Pain and trouble will come my way again. I'll fight my way down the Bitter Creek rapids again. But, the light in me will continue to shine. I don't fear the darkness ahead. I survived the darkness behind. Quietly knowing this will always light my way.

The Dance

The Cork

A few years ago, my family and I spent a day at the Indiana Dunes National Lakeshore. We arrived at the beach just as the sun rose and Lake Michigan was smooth with hardly a wave. Sitting in the sand with my feet in the cool water, I picked up a flat stone and tried to make it skip on the lake. It sank like, well... a rock. I tried again and the same thing happened. Meanwhile, Steve threw rocks and they skipped six, seven, nine times before sinking. Frustrated, I called, "How are you doing that?"

"It's all in how you throw it." Steve flipped a little rock and it skipped eleven times.

I tossed a rock. Plop! Tried again. Nope. When Steve finished laughing at me, he taught me how to skip rocks. A flick of the wrist, and a little practice later, I skipped rocks on the water. Steve and I hunted in the sand for flat rocks and tried to see who could skip one the farthest. He usually won, but I didn't mind.

As the sun rose higher in the sky, Lake Michigan woke up grumpy. We couldn't skip rocks anymore. Waves hit the little stones and down they went.

Before I landed in Nightmare Creek, I think I skipped through life like a stone on a calm lake. Dodging trouble here and there, full of life and boundless energy, I just skipped along happily. Until life's waves hit me, and I sank. I wrestled and fought my way back to the shore. When life calmed down, I skipped along happily again. This worked fine until I got dumped in Nightmare Creek.

For a long time, the current tossed me under water, and I fought to find my way back to the shore. Once I realized I was never getting back to the shore, I had to find a way to rise above. I had to become like a cork.

Unlike rocks, corks obviously float. They may sink a little, but they always find their way back up. Waves can toss corks around, but they keep right on floating no matter what. After I put aside the anger and frustration, I learned to quit struggling against the current in Nightmare Creek and just float. Not in bitter resignation, but in quiet acceptance. However, acceptance isn't the only thing keeping me bobbing like a cork.

Just because I have a serious illness doesn't mean I have to be serious. It's not like me to be serious for very long. If I'm invited to stay at a friend's house, you can guarantee I'll pack a hairdryer in my luggage and ask where I can plug it in. Or I'll pretend to panic at the airport because I didn't bring a hair brush!

I might look like a grownup, but really I'm an oversized kid. Playing around comes naturally to me. Did you know I want a purple wig? I want to draw on purple eyebrows to match my new purple hair. Hey, people stare at me all the time. Might as well give 'em something to look at.

I laugh a lot. When my body zigs when it should zag, I laugh. I have the weirdest problems doing the most basic things. Sometimes I can chew, but can't swallow. So, I end up with food in my mouth and no where for it to go.

Wait two minutes.

OK, now I can swallow, but I can't chew anymore.

Wait two more minutes.

Great, I can chew and swallow. Yay! Except, I can't move my arms, so I can't pick up a spoon. How ridiculous is that? No wonder it makes me laugh.

The summer of 2005, I was in a restaurant and I ordered an ice cream sundae. At the time, MG almost eliminated my ability to chew and swallow. I didn't order nuts on my sundae, so figured I could eat it. It was soft and required no chewing. Boy, was I wrong!

Fumbling with the long spoon, I scooped up some whipped cream and put it in my mouth. All of the muscles in my mouth simultaneously said, "What am I supposed to do with this fluffy goop?"

Instead of directing the whipped cream toward the back of my mouth, my weak tongue pushed it forward into my upper lip. Whipped cream melted into a puddle and spilled out of my mouth like a fountain. I could not stop laughing! The sheer weirdness of MG cracks me up.

I laugh at the absurd and unexpected challenges MG gives me. Then again, sometimes, I laugh because my only other alternative is tears. I've heard the saying, "When life gives you lemons, make lemonade." What about when life gives you onions? See, in my life I've got an awful lot of onions and not a lemon in sight. I've never heard of onion-ade.

When life gives you onions, you're gonna cry. The morning chemo made my hair fall out, I stood in front of the mirror and bawled. Pulling out hair and sobbing, I thought I'd never laugh again.

Finally, I reached for a tissue and dried my eyes. Stuck on the tissue were little black eyelashes and eyebrows. The paperwork from my oncologist said to expect hair loss. "Hair loss may include scalp, facial and body hair."

Wait! Hold on! Facial hair is a man's beard, not my eyebrows and eyelashes! But, there on the tissue were eyebrow hairs and eyelashes. I remember staring at them and saying, "You've gotta be kidding me!" Then I laughed so hard I had to lie down.

I think when life gives me onions, I end up laughing just because the situation is so outrageous and bizarre, it's funny. Laughing protects my heart from despair.

Having a chronic illness feels like getting in a limousine dressed for a night on the town and arriving at the base of a sheer mountain, instead. Without a word, the driver drops you off in the middle of nowhere and drives away. Wearing heels and a little black dress, you have to go mountain climbing. You have no survival gear, no ropes, no experience, and no guide. Aw. Too bad. You're on your own. Go up.

If that actually happened, first you would panic. Then you'd get angry. Next you'd collapse in a huge emotional meltdown. And then, when there's absolutely nothing else left to do, you'd laugh. How silly is rock climbing in heels? It's impossible. And yet, that's exactly what living with a chronic illness feels like.

Every day I'm asked to do the impossible, even if it is something as ordinary as eating whipped cream. After the panic, rage, and teary meltdowns, laughter is all that's left. When everything goes wrong, laughter is my sanity preserving safety valve. If I couldn't laugh, I wouldn't have the strength to stay alive. The trouble in my life would overwhelm me and sink me like a stone. Keeping my sense of humor is a priority for me. When I laugh, I rise above and keep floating like a cork in Lake Michigan.

Oops!
(For Dorothy Lund, my favorite cello teacher)

Imagine you're watching a movie, and two characters had a huge fight. While they're talking it over and working it out, which instrument is playing in the background? More often than not, it's the cello. What about when the hero dies tragically? Which instrument is wailing mournfully? Yup, it's the cello.

Able to sing in the same range as the human voice, the cello is an expressive, emotionally powerful instrument. In the movies, composers often choose the cello for deeply emotional scenes.

My personal favorite on-screen cello moment is in the middle of *The Lord of the Rings: The Return of the King*. It's during the siege of the city of Gondor. Pippin is afraid that he's going to die. Then Gandalf gently talks to Pippin about life after death. In the background, cellos softly sing *Into the West*. Ah. Love that scene! Had to be the cello singing. Just wouldn't have worked with a ukulele.

It takes hundreds of lessons, and thousands of hours practicing, to play any instrument well. However, fully expressing the poignant, voice like quality of the cello

115

calls for something beyond talent, beyond technique, even beyond practicing. To convey emotion through a cello, emotional sensitivity must live inside the cellist. My cellist friends and I jokingly call the expressive, emotional parts of ourselves our, "cello personalities."

People with cello personalities feel the full range of emotions to their zenith. When life is good, we're dancing. When life is difficult, we get as melancholy as a cello can sing. You don't even want to know what happens when we get angry!

Cellists are capable of belly laughter and crying meltdowns in the same afternoon, sometimes within the span of five minutes. In fact, it's not unusual for a cellist to cry during a Hallmark commercial. If you think I'm kidding, watch TV with me sometime.

Cellists have to be emotionally sensitive, or we would play the notes with all the warmth and depth of a computer. It's a passionate instrument and passionate people play it. Like a plug in a socket, our emotions give our cellos power.

I was nine when I started playing the cello. I do not clearly remember life before I had a cello in my arms, except for this: I remember feeling emotions I couldn't understand, or express, until I got my first, half-sized, plywood cello.

From the earliest hours with my miniature cello in Mrs. Lund's living room, I understood it was my voice. My cello sings what my words cannot say. My cello personality is one of my greatest treasures and I celebrate it every day.

Studying classical music gave me a rock solid foundation as a musician. I've played everything from Bach to Stravinsky. I've performed in many orchestras. I've even played under Sir Georg Solti, the legendary conductor of the Chicago Symphony Orchestra. I've had many amazing adventures with my cello.

However, the rigorous training classical music demanded, taught me more than technique. Combined with my cello personality, I learned to tear myself apart.

When practicing a concerto, there was the right way to play the music, and what I was playing. I knew what I wanted to hear, but I wasn't doing it right. What I was playing wasn't good enough. Practice the same 12 note passage over and over for an hour. Five hours. Nine hours later, that 12 note passage was still not good enough. Fingers throbbing, nails separating from my nail beds, I kicked myself without mercy. "What's wrong with me! I must suck at the cello."

In various practice rooms, I've shredded myself, picked up the pieces, and shoved them in the shredder again until there was only dust left behind. One thing I didn't do was laugh.

Overwhelmed by the gap between what I expected from myself, and what I was doing, I felt like a failure. No matter how hard I tried, I couldn't live up to my expectations.

Then MG changed everything. My whole life exploded on impact. Questions I never imagined asking became a regular part of my day. Can I walk over there? Can I eat that? Can I pick that up? How am I going to move this? Am I strong enough to open the door? OK, my mouth is full of toothpaste foam and I can't spit it out. What do I do now?

MG battered me beyond anything I could have imagined, literally beyond recognition. The jagged rocks and swift current of Nightmare Creek changed my appearance. The scar on my chest is more than cosmetic. Beneath it my bones still ache. I got the hiccups tonight and my collarbones are sore right now.

Chest surgery left me fragile inside and out. Days later, I was amazed I could be so shattered and still be alive. Recovering from surgery forced me to treat myself gently. Survival demanded going slowly, one baby step at a time. If I rushed something, like the first time I lifted my cello, my body let me know I'd made a mistake. I had to tune in to my body, really listen to what she was telling me.

The lessons I learned during the University of Catastrophe class, *Surviving a Sternotomy*, I still carry with me. I learned I'm not invincible and I have limits. I have physical limits, like how far I can walk.

I have emotional limits, like choosing not to watch frightening movies. I don't need to see gory images of a pretend electric saw cutting someone open. I've survived a real electric saw cutting me open.

Surviving surgery taught me to respect my limits. It taught me to treat myself more gently. My body isn't perfect, and neither am I. Instead of beating myself up for a mistake, I stop and take a deep breath. I remind myself life beats me up enough. It doesn't need any help from me.

I've learned mistakes don't mean I'm a failure. I've survived too much, and come too far, to be a failure. Instead of getting down on myself when I make mistakes, I try to learn from them. That's all I can ask of myself.

I'm slowly learning to balance my expectations with reality. Gone are the nine hour marathon practice sessions that brought more tears than triumph. MG limits how my arms and hands move, limits how I can move around my cello.

I'll never have the technical skill of a master cellist. But, I can still play. I've worked very hard to keep my cello in my arms and instead of beating myself up for every mistake, I cherish singing with my cello. I can still sing from my spirit. That is better than good enough.

When I was in orchestra, conductors often said, "If you're gonna make a mistake, make a loud one." A loud mistake let conductors know what we needed to work on in rehearsal, not what needed to be judged. Rehearsing music and making mistakes go together like peanut butter and jelly. Truth is, everyone who plays music makes mistakes. I'm a grand champion at them.

On stage, with only one shot at it, the likelihood of my blowing something goes up exponentially. A few years ago, I was playing ten Christmas concerts and I messed up the same note in *O Come All Ye Faithful* at all ten shows. It wasn't a solo. I was one of a group of cellists, in a full orchestra, plus a choir, and the audience was singing along. The music was so loud the conductor didn't know I goofed up, neither did the audience, but I knew.

Now, this wasn't a hard note to play. It was one of the notes I learned to play during my earliest cello lessons with Mrs. Lund in 1978. There is no logical reason why I blew it ten times. I've played the same note perfectly thousands and thousands of times. I guess it's one of those Murphy's laws of music: the easier it is to play, the more likely Marie will screw it up!

I marked the note in my music in pencil, and then with a star around it. I even put an arrow by it in purple marker. In rehearsal, I played the music perfectly. During every show, right before we played that Christmas carol, I'd whisper to my stand partner, "OK, I'm gonna get it right this time."

I was playing along beautifully and then, *honk!* Sounded dreadful. We'd fight back a giggle fit and somehow keep playing. But, after my tenth screw up, my stand partner and I laughed so hard we almost had to leave the stage!

During those concerts I failed to play one note right. One note among hundreds. There was a time when I would have beaten myself to a pulp over that. I'd have decided I wasn't good enough. But, now I know it's not worth the energy to panic over a bobbled note. Since I figured that out, I've had a lot more fun playing my cello.

Mistakes are part of life. Big ones and small ones, even cello ones. Accepting myself, even when I make a mistake, is easier now because I know my strengths. Fighting MG has taught me who I am, and who I am not. I am very comfortable with myself, aware of where I fail and succeed. A mistake doesn't threaten my strengths, doesn't negate them in any way. So, I can lighten up when things go wrong.

The Shield

At The University of Catastrophe I learned to treat myself gently when I made a mistake. In elementary school, I learned the exact opposite lesson. When I was a kid, my mistakes were funny for everyone, but me. Mess up a math problem on the chalkboard, kids laughed. Trip over a jump rope and fall on the playground, kids laughed. Misspell a word during a spelling bee, strikeout in softball, spill my milk on my shirt during lunch, kids laughed.

It wasn't only mistakes that made the kids in my class laugh. Weigh more than the other kids, talk differently, walk differently, any little difference, kids laughed. In elementary school, I learned being different was shameful. I learned to hide anything about me that was different so I could fit in. Kids who couldn't hide their differences were shunned. If they were lucky, shunning was the only thing that happened to them. Some kids at my school were chum surrounded by sharks.

At my school, the ultimate sign of being different was riding a little school bus. Anyone who came to school on a little bus went to different classes than me. They were in special ed, a mysterious area of my school I heard about but never actually saw.

The special ed classes had gym at a different time than us. They ate lunch in a different lunch room. During recess on the playground, we went inside as the special ed classes went out to play. We never played together.

My teachers scolded everyone for teasing the kids in special ed, but never encouraged us to say hello. Teachers didn't show me how to relate to someone who couldn't see, or couldn't hear, someone with a developmental delay, or someone using a wheelchair. But, just because I wasn't taught, doesn't mean I didn't learn. I learned they were different.

They were not... us.

Fast forward 25 years. I have many disabilities. I struggle to walk, talk, chew and swallow. If I was disabled like I am now, back in the 70's, I would have arrived at school on a little bus. I'd zip my powerchair past my old classroom to the special ed classroom. An occupational therapist would have helped me hold a spoon steady. A physical therapist would have helped me with my balance.

One thing wouldn't have happened. No one would have handed me a cello and encouraged me to play. I wouldn't have been included in orchestra rehearsals or talent shows. If you saw me drooling on my shirt right now, gifted cellist probably wouldn't come to mind.

Even though it bothers me, I'm judged by how I look. My physical limitations sometimes limit people's expectations of me. Sad as it is, just because I am comfortable with myself doesn't mean other people are comfortable around me.

The first thing people notice about me is I'm seated on a chair with wheels on it. Some people gape at me as if I'm riding a flying carpet. Other times, little kids stare at me and point. Their parents, apologizing profusely, quickly shoo them away.

Rowdy teens play chicken with my powerchair, thinking it's great fun to block me with their bicycles and bodies. The temptation to run over the loudest teen, in front of the girl he's trying to impress, runs through my mind. Remembering what a fool I was when I was a teen, I resist the temptation and keep right on cruising.

I understand completely why people stare at me. People are wired to notice something different and sort of blur over the familiar. There's survival value in noticing something is out of the ordinary. If there was a rattlesnake on your kitchen floor, noticing would keep you from getting bitten.

Since most people walk, someone cruising into a mall using a powerchair is going to get noticed. A bald chick cruising into the mall using a powerchair, is definitely gonna get noticed. Bald, using a powerchair, with a dog beside me, anonymity is not an option. Might as well have a neon flashing sign saying, "Here I come! Look at me!"

This is when my sense of humor becomes a shield for me. Instead of getting offended when people stare, I laugh inside. Laughing reminds me that I'm OK. All of the negative lessons I learned on the playground I'm slowly overcoming. In school, I learned being different was shameful. All of the stares and pitying looks, rude comments, and averted gazes, remind me that some people still feel that way.

I'm not struggling to be normal. I am normal. The way my body functions, and doesn't function, is normal for me. The attitude that I must somehow make up for my disabilities, and overcome them, is baloney. I cannot overcome what MG has done. All I can do is be me.

Being me means laughing. It means enjoying music on my iPod while cooking dinner for my family. Being me means enjoying beer and football with Steve Sunday afternoons, and groaning when the Bears quarterback throws another interception. It means enjoying sci-fi movies, especially anything with *Godzilla* in the title. After a bad day, there is something healing about watching a rubber monster destroy Tokyo. Run for your lives, everybody! It's Godzilla!

Being me means putting little treasures in a box and mailing a box o' fun to someone I love. Being me means loving the people I care about openly, and receiving their love back, just as openly. Being me means enjoying a glass of red wine at the end of a long day.

Most of the time I forget about being disabled and concentrate on enjoying life. Able bodied or disabled, I treat people the way I'd like to be treated: like they're normal, because they are normal and OK. Some people I meet may never be completely comfortable around me. That's all right. Their stares and pitying looks can't get past my shield of laughter. I'm me in here and I like being me just fine.

The Perfect Patsy

The day this happened, I freely admit I was in a goofy mood. Full of mischief, waiting for an opportunity to let my inner prankster loose, all I needed was a perfect patsy to play with. I was in the store with my service dog by my side, when Patsy walked up to me. I don't think that was the woman's name, but that's what I'm going to call her because poor Patsy walked up to me at the wrong time, on the wrong day. What followed was a conversation I'll never forget.

I was in the cereal aisle, buying Lucky Charms for Evelyn, when Pasty said, "I just have to tell you, I think you're such an inspiration."

Startled, I looked up and saw a woman roughly in her fifties. Since she was smiling, I realized she was trying to pay me a complement. Telling me I'm inspiring, when I'm not doing anything inspiring, irritates me. It irritates my friend, Lee, too.

Lee is inspiring when she helps a customer at the Chicago Lighthouse. Her compassion, patience and knowledge is inspiring. Lee is not inspiring when she eats an ice cream cone while visually impaired.

I'm not inspiring while cereal shopping, either. I'm just a mom buying breakfast cereal with the nutritional value of sugar cubes, because Evelyn cleaned the kitchen without complaining every day for a week.

If I was in a normal mood, I might have said, "Thank you," and rolled away from Patsy feeling embarrassed and slighted.

However, I was definitely not in a normal mood! I was... How can I explain? We used to have a cat named, Teaspoon. We named her Teaspoon because when she was a kitten, she was a mere teaspoon full of a cat. Anyhow, when Teaspoon caught a mouse she always toyed with it until it died of exhaustion. Sometimes, it took hours. Just like Tom and Jerry cartoons, Teaspoon would corner the mouse. Let it go. Corner it again. Nibble nibble. Ooh, you squealed. Poor thing. Think I'll let you go. The frightened mouse scurried away. Psych! You're mine.

I gotta tell you that I used to feel bad for the mouse. Until I realized the mouse was the dummy who picked the house with the cat. Darwin the Mouse, your clueless genes will not be passed on to future generations.

Up until I met Patsy, I had no idea how much joy Teaspoon felt when she played with mice. I get it now.

After Patsy said I was inspiring, I looked up at her and asked, "Why do you think I'm inspiring?"

"Because..." she appeared flustered by the question.

Good.

"Um, I think people like you are very inspiring."

"People with freckles and glasses?" I asked innocently.

"No. People like you." She gestured toward my wheelchair and dog.

"My wheelchair makes me inspiring?"

"Yes. I see you here shopping all the time and you're always happy. You used to walk and now… I just think that's so inspiring, considering your infirmity."

What? I almost fell out of my chair. Did Patsy just say infirmity? I think she did. Letting that one go, I gave her my best puzzled look. "I'm inspiring because I'm using a wheelchair and having a good day? Why is that inspiring?"

Patsy furrowed her brow. This conversation wasn't turning out the way she planned. Clearly uncomfortable, she said, "I just meant…"

I cut her off. "You meant that it's inspiring to you when you see a person in a wheelchair doing something ordinary. My question is, why is that inspiring?"

After a moment, Patsy said, "Because if I was all crippled up…"

No, I am not making that up! The woman actually said, "all crippled up." And I thought *infirmity* was gonna make me fall out of my chair. I bit my cheek so hard to keep from laughing, I still have a scar inside my mouth.

"… I couldn't be happy."

OK. I hear this way too often. Why does a wheelchair symbolize the end of happiness? On an ordinary day, the pissed-off-o-meter would have hit the red zone. That day? Oh, I was having way too much fun. "You wouldn't be happy?" I repeated, sounding sad. "How come?"

"Because… because everything would be so diffi-cult."

"Some things are difficult, but…" I reached into the basket on my lap and dropped a bottle of shampoo on the floor. My service dog jumped to her feet, grabbed the bottle and put it in my hand. "I find ways around it."

Patsy said, "Your dog is beautiful."

"Thank you. Honey makes my life easier."

"I'll bet. How long have you been confined to a wheelchair?"

Oops. Patsy just stepped in it again! "Confined?" I rolled my chair forward and back. Honey did a cha-cha beside me. "Do I look confined?" Wrestling back hysterical laughter, I said, "I was confined before I got a wheelchair. Now I'm not confined. I can go anywhere I want."

"Sorry. I meant wheelchair bound."

Oh poor Patsy! I looked at my lap and around my wheelchair. "Bound? I don't see any duct tape or ropes."

"That's not what I meant, I meant…"

"You meant wheelchair user. Bound and confined make it sound like my chair is a trap. My wheelchair lets me go anywhere I want to go. I'm seated in a chair. Not trapped by it."

Pasty smiled at me. "I never really thought about it that way. Wow! I learned a lot from you. Thanks for talk-ing to me."

"You're welcome." I rolled away thinking, thanks for being the perfect Patsy!

Joy Benchmarks

Today is a good day. However, my definition of a good day might be different from yours. Just like how dark midnight looks depends on where you are. If you're standing outside a casino in Vegas, midnight might not look very dark. If you're in suburban Chicago, it's dark enough to see a few stars. However, midnight in rural Michigan where I used to live is really dark.

My house was a mile from the nearest neighbor, isolated deep in the woods. If I forgot to leave the porch light on, it was dark enough to walk past my own house. Been there. Done that. Felt really dumb. I loved living in the woods. Turn off the light and it was pitch black at night. Living there gave me a whole new benchmark for dark as midnight.

Because of what I've lived through, I have a whole new set of benchmarks for what a good day looks like, too. Did today involve the word, "scan?" No? Then today is a good day. Did today involve the word, "surgery?" No? Then today is a good day. When I sat down with a bowl of chocolate ice cream, could I eat it? Yes? Then today is a very good day.

Without the grief of having multiple ultrasounds, MRI and CT scans, not having a scan today would hardly be a reason to smile. Since I've been scanned so often it's a wonder I don't have super powers, or glow in the dark, not having a scan today makes me happy.

Not having to wait for test results makes me happy, too. Had I never experienced the hurt of a thymoma, not having cancer wouldn't be a reason for laughter. After all, most people don't have cancer right now, and they don't celebrate being cancer free, either. Not having cancer is something most people take for granted. Want to know how awesome not having cancer is? Just ask a cancer survivor. They'll tell you. How good is it to be able to eat ice cream? Considering I couldn't swallow ice cream six months ago, and I can now, it's wonderful.

It doesn't take much to make me happy. Being alive makes me happy. Meanwhile, companies spend millions of dollars on advertising trying to convince me their products will make me happy. Marie will not be happy until she owns our cell phone. She won't be satisfied until she eats our hamburger. She won't be beautiful until she uses our skin cream. Life without our widget will not be happy. I used to believe it. Then I got sick and I got a whole new outlook. Now I know what really matters to me isn't on sale at Wal-mart.

Walking short distances makes me happy. Wheelchairs make me happy, too. Wheelchairs let me do things I couldn't do if I had to walk. I love the balance I have between walking and wheeling. I am blessed I can stand up long enough to hug someone I love. Then I can sit down and not have to worry about getting too tired.

A casual stroll by a mountain stream with a friend, makes me happy. Sitting in front of the fireplace with my husband and daughter, while our two dogs, Honey and April, snuggle with us, makes me happy. I love making up a new song on my cello just because I can. I enjoy the simple pleasures in life just because I can.

Simple pleasures aren't small to me at all. I've been too sick to sit in a wheelchair. I know how it feels to live in a bed, too sick to even sit by the fire with my family. I enjoy simple pleasures more deeply now than before I got sick. Sorrow reset my joy benchmarks.

For a time, the hole in me was filled with bitterness and anger. Then tears washed the anger away. Once I reached beyond the hurt, I discovered joy benchmarks are a matter of perspective.

A pocket sized flashlight on the strip in Vegas won't help you find your hotel. You probably won't even notice the light. In rural Michigan, a pocked sized flashlight meant the difference between getting home or sleeping under a pine tree. When I forgot to leave the porch light on, my little flashlight meant everything to me.

The darker the road, the more precious light becomes. Since I've walked down a terrible dark road, I can celebrate the tiniest rays of light in my life. I have joy benchmarks that many people don't have, and I treasure them all.

Can I see the vivid red cardinal standing in the snow? Yes. Then stop everything and look at it. Stop and celebrate eyes that see. Can I eat today? Yes. Then stop and savor the taste of chocolate ice cream. I remember what it felt like to eat tears instead of ice cream.

Thanks to the chemo, I can eat again. I can chew and swallow everything I like to eat. I don't cook meals for my family, and then watch them eat, feeling hungry and left out. Last night I ate chicken casserole with my family, and was truly thankful for the food and their company. Eating ice cream right now is reminding me that eating is a gift. Just like fighting for my life reminds me that life is a gift.

Perhaps my new joy benchmarks are the greatest reward from sticking it out at The University of Catastrophe. I take less for granted and celebrate life more. Deep loss has taught me to love the people around me more powerfully. It has helped me feel their love more powerfully as well.

With my joy benchmarks set on low, I savor life's little treasures. Chocolates. Sandhill cranes in flight. Cookies baking in the oven. Cello strings vibrating under my fingers. My daughter Evelyn laughing with her dad in the living room. These are the things I celebrate, the things that really matter.

I'm discovering the lazy pace of life up Nightmare Creek makes it easier for me to stop and notice, stop and celebrate. I'm outside of the hustle and bustle with time to be still. People feel sorry for me because I'm sick from the chemo right now. Recovering from chemo is tough, true. But, I don't think it's as tough as being too busy to notice a red cardinal in the snow. I'm watching one hop around right now. When I press my nose against a frost covered window just to watch a cardinal, I remember my joy benchmarks and feel so satisfied I wouldn't change a thing.

Angel

In the summer of 2002, I decided I wanted a puppy. Unfortunately, Steve made it very clear he didn't want a dog – not that something as minor as my husband's opinion was going to stop me. Roughly every thirty seconds, if my husband was in earshot, I whined about needing a puppy.

"But, puppies are so soft!"

"Puppies are so cute!"

"Puppies are so cuddly and sweet!"

Steve tried to convince me that we had cats and didn't need a dog. He even offered to buy me a new kitten. Obviously that wasn't going to work. All I wanted was a puppy. As July turned to August, August turned to September, and September turned to October, Steve realized nothing short of a real live puppy was going to shut me up. He's stubborn, not stupid.

On October 19, 2002, Steve caved. He brought me to the pet store to look at the puppies. In the parking lot, he reminded me *twice* that we were only going to look at the puppies and definitely not getting one. Uh-huh. In a big black bin with cedar chips on the bottom was a litter of

Labrador retriever and German shepherd mutts. They'd been in the store a total of three hours.

Some of the pups were black and tan. Some were yellow and cream. All of them were adorable. Evelyn, Steve, and I, each picked out a yellow puppy and started cooing at it. Of the three, the puppy in Steve's arms was the calmest. He passed the puppy to me. When the fat little puppy licked the tip of my nose, it was all over.

The puppy's left front foot had tiny spots on it like she splashed in a puddle of honey. Those golden spots, plus her honey gold little ears, is how Honey got her name.

Actually, that's not even remotely true. It sounded plausible, but I just lied. Sorry about that. Embarrassing as this is, right after Steve handed me the calm little puppy, I feverishly squeaked at her, "Oh, honey! Oh, honey! Oh, honey! Oh honey!"

Steve grinned and said, "That's a good name for the dog."

Dummy me, I asked, "What is?"

"Oh, Honey! Oh Honey!" Steve said, teasing me. So, that's how Honey got her name.

On the way home, Steve and Evelyn made fun of me for sounding like a total fool in the store, but I didn't care. Besides, the joke is on Steve. Not only did Mister, "We aren't getting a dog no matter how much you whine about it," pick out my puppy, he named her, too! So, I got the last laugh, and my new puppy.

Needless to say, I was beside myself that afternoon, reveling in honey and cream colored furry delight. Eight-weeks-old and illegally cute, Honey quickly became my new shadow. Honey spent just about every waking moment in my arms. When I wasn't carting her around, I snuggled with Honey on the couch. I pretended I was bonding with my new friend. In reality I was indulging in the spoils of war. Months of hard cajoling, whining, fawning and scraping paid off. I had my puppy and absolutely no clue what to do next.

Up until I had a puppy, I thought housebreaking meant trying to teach the puppy to pee and poop outside. What was I thinking? Housebreaking is what a puppy does as soon as *you* go to the bathroom. In the time it takes an average person to use the toilet, wash hands and return to the kitchen, a puppy can eat a sponge mop, piddle a gallon, chew a hole in the back door, pull threads out of a rug, and destroy a whole roll of paper towels. Imagine a toddler with teeth and warp speed, and that pretty much sums up what Honey was like. She was terrible!

I think I had Honey a total of two weeks when I realized one of us was going to be trained. I assumed it was going to be the dog. I was wrong.

First I trained myself to sleep fully clothed with my shoes beside my bed, so I could take Honey outside in the middle of the night to snuffle leaves in the snow, but not pee. I also trained myself to chase Honey away from the cats she found so fascinating.

Stalking cats was Honey's favorite game. Until Sanka, our elderly black cat, had enough of that and hissed at Honey and chased her from room to room. Honey gave Sanka plenty of space after that. Watching a puppy three times the size of a cat dart in terror isn't something I'll soon forget.

As far as Honey was concerned, housebreaking was going well by the time she was four-months-old. She already destroyed a rug, a hundred pens, several shoes, two mops and my sanity. That was when the most unexpected thing happened.

In early January 2003, I sat at my desk while Honey busied herself with yanking off my socks. I bobbled a blue pen. The pen tumbled off the chair arm and landed within two inches of my pen munching puppy. I imagined cleaning ink and Bic bits off of the rug again.

Before I had a chance to reach down and get the pen, the inevitable happened. She snatched my pen in her teeth. Then Honey did the most unlikely thing imaginable. She lifted up her soft fuzzy head and gently placed the pen in the palm of my hand. With her tender brown eyes, Honey said, *Here you go, Mama. You dropped this.* Then Honey sat at my feet.

Pen in hand, I gaped at the strange puppy blinking up at me, and wondered what she did with Honey! In that moment a light bulb went off in my mind. If Honey could, without any training at all, pick up a pen and hand it to me, what could she be trained to do? Instantly, Honey's life changed and so did mine. My new friend became my service dog in training.

The moment Honey picked up my pen and put it in my hand, she decided to become my service dog. It truly was her decision. Oddly enough, it never occurred to me to get a service dog, let alone train one. When I got Honey,

I thought I was getting a new friend. I never dreamed I would get so much more.

Now, I knew nothing about training my own service dog, so I enrolled Honey in dog obedience class. Since Honey showed such an amazing aptitude for disobedience, I had no idea what to expect. I needn't have worried. Honey adored the training ring. From her first class, Honey saw people were watching her and she fell in love.

The first week, the trainers told us to heel our dogs around the ring. Honey strutted around the ring with her tail up and chest out. Honey quickly became a favorite with the trainers. A few weeks later, we were supposed to practice getting our dogs to come to us from six feet away. One of the trainers decided to use Honey as a demo dog.

I handed over the leash. The trainer told Honey to sit. Honey sat upright and perfectly. Then the trainer said, "Come!" Honey ran straight to the trainer in a direct bee line and sat. Everyone in the training ring laughed.

"OK, your dog doesn't have to sit," the trainer said, shaking her head. "Let me try that again." The trainer tried it a second time. Honey came toward the trainer even faster and sat perfectly even with the woman's feet like a champion obedience dog. I remember watching my dog and just laughing. Whatever I asked of Honey, she did, usually far exceeding expectations. Training her was so effortless, I felt like I was cheating.

Now, I've got to tell you, Steve noticed I was having fun training my dog and he got jealous. So, Steve got himself a weimaraner puppy and named her, April. Having two puppies at the same time meant tag team trouble, and doubled our laughter. But, soon both of our dogs were enrolled in obedience classes and both dogs did well.

Every day Honey and I practiced obedience exercises. Week after week, Honey kept doing better and better. When Honey was 13-months-old, I decided if she was going to be a service dog, she needed proof of obedience training. So, I decided to take her through the American Kennel Club Canine Good Citizen test.

This test showcases how well a dog follows basic commands like sit, lie down, stay and come. Also, they test how the dog reacts to noise, other dogs and strangers.

I was nervous the day of the test. Wearing an arm band, placed in an unfamiliar training ring, I didn't know how Honey would do. Would she notice she was only wearing a buckle collar instead of her training collar? Would Honey notice I didn't have any treats in my pockets? Would she pass or fail?

Again, I didn't need to worry. Honey passed the entire test with flying colors her first time through. In less than a year, I went from having a wild puppy destroying my house, to having a trained dog with the papers to prove it. Now all I needed to do was train Honey to perform service dog tasks to help me, and we would be all set, right?

Wrong.

Devil

(For Evelyn, who loves to laugh)

When Honey was 13-months-old, she graduated from obedience school. Because I'm weird, my dog has photographs of herself wearing a black mortar board and a black gown marking her graduation. My dog is trained. No one has to take my word for it. I have a diploma from the American Kennel Club certifying that my dog is a trained Canine Good Citizen.

You know something else? I have a diploma from my junior high school. It's a fancy piece of paper stating I learned everything I was supposed to learn in junior high. But, I swear all I learned in junior high was how to shoot rubber bands off of my braces with my tongue.

All of the paperwork I have from grammar school to college certifies I learned certain things long enough to repeat them correctly on the right test, on the right day. Fancy diplomas don't mean much for humans, and dogs it turns out.

Literally the next day after Honey earned her Canine Good Citizen award, I took her to the park where we always trained. Just like always, I said, "Honey, sit."

My AKC certified trained dog looked at me with her brown eyes wide, and did... nothing. Honey stood there, looking me directly in the eye and did not sit.

But, I swear I heard her whisper, *Um, you know, I've thought about it and decided it's against my religious principles to sit on wet grass.*

"Honey, sit."

And also on wet pavement. That is strictly taboo.

Convinced there was some kind of miscommunication going on, I asked her to sit a third time. "Honey, sit!"

My dog laughed at me. *Sit? Oh, you mean I should sit. . . now? Here? Are you crazy? I heard a story from Butterscotch, the lab who lives around the corner, that there was a sheltie who sat in this exact spot on the grass, and he was abducted by aliens. You wouldn't want that to happen to me, would you? So, you see, I can't possibly sit. Try asking me to lie down.*

I gave up on asking her to sit and moved on with our training routine. "Honey, down."

You obviously don't want me to lie down. Not here. Hello? Aliens? Abduction? Does that ring a bell?

"Honey, down."

Wait a sec, Mama. Down. Really? You want me to race down to the pond and nab a duck? That's the only thing you've said that made any sense. Great! I can do that. Uh, how come we're not racing toward the pond like we're supposed to? I thought you wanted a duck.

Picture me in the park absolutely flabbergasted. I gaped at the strange dog blinking up at me, wondering what she did with Honey. It felt like someone else's dog was attached to my leash. Instead of sweet, compliant, certified Canine Good Citizen, Honey, I had a totally un-trained dog in front of me. This strange dog, who looked exactly like Honey, just stood there laughing at me.

Frustrated, I asked Honey, "What's wrong with you? You did it perfectly yesterday!" Using my sternest dog trainer voice, I said, "Honey, that's enough! Down!"

Down. Down. I used to know what that meant. Give me a minute. Um. . . down. Duck down! That's right! There are ducks to chase. C'mon, let's chase ducks.

I gave up, and decided to work on something easy. "Honey, heel."

Honey did not move. She snickered at me. *I'm a dog. I'm not licensed to practice medicine. Duh!*

Just like in dog class, I moved forward and tugged Honey with me. Sharply, I said, "Honey, heel!"

She suddenly lunged forward as if we were in the Iditarod. Ever have a dog drag you into an evergreen bush? Hurts slightly less than being yanked head first into an apple tree. Brushing apple tree sticks out of my hair, and hanging on for dear life, I shouted, "No! Heel!"

Oh, OK, I'll march beside you until we get closer to the ducks. Then, whamo, I'm nabbing one of them critters.

Arm aching, I quit trying to make Honey walk with me and just said, "Honey, stay."

That's your cue, Mama. Drop the leash. That's it. Drop the leash and I'll go chase them ducks. Wait a sec. No fair! You didn't drop the leash! What gives?

I was wondering the exact same thing. What hap-pened to my obedient, perfect, easy to train, puppy? She passed her obedience exam the night before! Completely demoralized, I returned home and let Honey loose in the backyard to play. Maybe running around with April, and the neighborhood dogs, would knock some sense into her. At least I hoped it would. I was, of course, wrong.

"Honey, come!"

Yeah, right. Squirrels to chase. Flying plastic bags lofting on the breeze. Leaves fluttering on the grass. My friends are all out running around. And you want me to leave all this joy for a hunk of cheese and a pat on the head? Uh, yeah. Like that'll ever happen. You need therapy, Mama!

"Honey, come. Right now!"

"Run run as fast as you can, you can't catch me I'm the gingerbread man!" You really should consider therapy. It might help.

OK, at that point I was really mad. "Honey! Get over here!"

I'm coming, I'm coming. But. . . I'll move toward you extra slow, just because I can. Ooh, clover! I love how clover flowers smell. I'm going to sniff all 197 of them, one at a time, and then I'll come. You seem stressed. Therapy, Mama. I'll have the vet recommend someone for you.

Was Honey having an off day? No. Was I a bad dog trainer? No. Then what happened to Honey? What could change her from an angel to a devil in one day? Simple. Go into any animal shelter and I can guarantee you will find dogs between the ages of nine months and two and a half.

Why? Because people bring home a cute puppy not realizing it will turn into a willful, obnoxious teenager. Depending on the breed, the teenage phase can last months, or a year or more. A lot of new dog owners don't know that. So they take their unbearable teenage dog to the shelter, instead of going to a training class. A training class would let them know their teenage dog was being normal. Obnoxious, but normal.

Dog training classes didn't train my dog. They trained me. Class taught me how to command my dog, how to carry myself around my dog, so she would listen to me. Every week, my dog trainer said, "There can be only one alpha bitch in your house, Marie, and you'd better make sure it's you!"

Once Honey became a teenager, she tried to take my position as alpha bitch in the family pack. My eager to please puppy grew up. The diploma from the AKC we earned might as well have been written on toilet paper. My dog didn't respect me, listen to me, or even recognize I existed. Honey's teenage year was a nightmare, and one of the greatest joys of my life, all at the same time.

When Honey was small, I was Honey's friend and she did what I asked because we were friends. Once Honey became a teenager, if I was going to keep my sanity, let alone raise a service dog, I had to get Honey to listen to me. That morning in the park, Honey let me know it was time to quit being her buddy and become her leader. As far as Honey was concerned, my name became, "She who must be obeyed."

As soon as Honey became a teenager, treats became harder to get and praise even tougher. I became a drill sergeant, barking out rapid fire commands, "Sit, down, stand, stay, heel, down, come, sit." There was no praise between commands and no sign that I was even pleased with Honey. The rule was, do what I say now, because I said it.

I had one treat in my left hand, but Honey had no idea which command would earn her the cookie and praise. So, she did all commands as fast as possible. I strung together fifteen or twenty commands without a single praise or treat just because I was in charge.

In doggie boot camp, we drilled on pure obedience for three hours a day, every day, for six months. I wanted Honey to know that *sit* means put your butt down in a mud puddle. *Down* means drop on your belly in snow covered gravel. *Heel* means get even with my left knee and move where I go, even if it's in a cha-cha. *Stay* means if God shows up on a cloud and calls your name, don't move until I release you. When I say *come*, if a volcano erupts, the earth quakes, and a tornado blows, you come to my side because I called. I am she who must be obeyed, and you have two choices, Honey. You can do it my way, or you can do it my way.

The drills taught my teenage dog two critical things. I was alpha bitch. Honey was not. Teenage Honey responded to doggie boot camp absolutely gloriously.

"Honey, sit."

Sitting, ma'am. My butt is on the ground, and my paws are even with your toes, ma'am.

"Honey down."

Yes, ma'am.

"Honey, stand."

Attention!

"Honey, heel."

A left, a left, a left, right, left!

"Honey, turn."

About face!

"Honey stay."

Yes, ma'am. Understood. I'll stay at my post until dismissed.

"Honey, jump."

Jumping, ma'am. How high, ma'am?

"Honey, come."

Ma'am, yes, ma'am! Double time, ma'am!

The same flair she had for obedience in the training ring returned. Tail up and wagging, Honey ran through my drills with joyful, driven, gusto.

One treat obedience drill is now our favorite game to play. Either with hand signals or words, Honey just loves the game. If I was training a pet, I think I would have done exactly the same thing. A well trained dog is a joy to live with. But, of course I wasn't training a pet.

Once Honey respected me, and obeyed my commands, we started working on service dog tasks and I watched Honey become the dog she was born to be.

Gift

Since myasthenia gravis weakens my hands, I drop small things easily. It's also hard for me to keep my balance when I reach down to pick up a pen or a quarter. As challenging as it was to train Honey to listen to me, teaching her to retrieve small items was a breeze.

It's amazing to watch a service dog open a cupboard and bring a soda to her handler, but training that task is easy. It took twenty minutes and cost me a quarter cup of liverwurst.

I put a Pepsi can in Honey's mouth and traded the soda can for a lick of liverwurst. After doing that a few times, I put the Pepsi can on the floor. Since trading the can got her liverwurst a second ago, Honey quickly picked up the can off the floor and put it in my hand. We repeated picking up the can off the floor for a while. When I could tell she had the concept, I abandoned the Pepsi can.

My next step was training Honey to yank open the cupboard with a tug. With the cupboard door open, I put the tug in Honey's mouth and traded the tug for a lick of liverwurst. Then I slowly shut the cupboard door in stages

151

so she had to pull the door open in exchange for liverwurst. Took about five minutes for Honey to consistently yank open the door to get a snack.

Then, I showed Honey the forgotten Pepsi and she worked on getting the Pepsi off the floor again. After alternating between opening the cupboard and getting a Pepsi off the floor, I showed Honey the Pepsi can, but I put it inside the cupboard and shut the door. I said nothing. Just waited.

It took half a second for Honey to figure out what to do. *Open the cupboard, grab the Pepsi, put it in Mama's hand.*

Honey's tail almost wagged off the first time she yanked open the cupboard and got the Pepsi for me. She was more excited than I was. I gave her twenty licks of liverwurst, hugs, kisses and lots of petting. My signal to Honey that she got it right is a cheerful, "Yay!" My dog lives for that. So do I. While Honey bounced, I kept giving snacks and saying, "Yay!"

I did it! I'm good! I'm so good! Honey danced around the kitchen, wiggling every inch of her body. *More! Mama! More! This is fun! This is great! I can do it! Again! Again!*

I put the Pepsi back in the cupboard and waited for Honey to retrieve it. Then I took one step back from the cupboard. Two steps. Three. Now I can be in a different room, and say, "Honey, go get me a Pepsi." On cue, Honey will trot through the house, open the cupboard door, get a Pepsi, and bring it back through the house to my hand. Rule number one with myasthenia gravis: energy conservation. By going to the kitchen for me, Honey conserves my energy.

I trained Honey to pick up everything from dollar bills to paper clips the exact same way I taught her to retrieve a Pepsi from a cupboard. In tiny steps, with snacks and praise, I trained Honey to help me function.

Honey is trained to retrieve anything I ask her to get and put it in my hand. She's also trained to help me find a safe place to sit down if I get too tired. Through our bonding and work together, Honey can alert me to weak muscles before I fall. But, if I do fall down, Honey is trained to stand rigid and let me use her shoulders and the floor to stand up. She's even trained to help me get off the toilet should my thigh muscles fail. Her tasks make my life possible and I cannot imagine life without Honey beside me.

Not only does Honey help me physically, she's an emotional comfort as well. Having Honey by my side helps me be more independent. If I can't get off the toilet by myself, asking my dog for help preserves my dignity. If I need help, my dog never says, "I'm busy. Can you wait a minute?" Even if I drop the same dollar bill five times, she never says, "Again?" Honey simply gets it for me again and again without judgment or comment. To Honey, I'm not needy. I'm just her partner and friend.

The work I put into training Honey built my self-confidence. Having my body fall apart shook my self-esteem. Things I used to do without thinking, like unloading the clothes dryer, became hard. It's hard to need help after years of independence. Since I was less capable of doing things, I felt less capable inside. My body changed me into someone I didn't want to become. I felt like a three headed alien when people stared at me. I became shy, re-clusive and unsure of myself. Going out into public wasn't worth it.

Training Honey required that I show leadership. To get Honey to respect me, I had to carry myself as someone worthy of respect. I had to speak with confidence, act with confidence, or she would ignore me.

To train Honey, I had to go into public places and be confident when I got there, so Honey would know I was still in charge. If someone challenged my civil right to bring my dog with me, I had to speak up for myself. Having Honey beside me forced me to be assertive instead of timid. I can honestly say, my dog brought out the best in me.

When I go into a store with Honey, people stare at the dog, not at me. Gazes are softened instead of averted. People come up to me all the time in stores to admire Honey. They ask questions about her. When I answer, I make eye contact instead of shying away. Then people tell me about their dogs. My wheelchair disappears. I become just another dog lover, chatting about dogs. I'm not the wheelchair lady anymore, but the lady with the cool helper dog who picks up dimes.

Now that Honey is trained, our partnership is like a ballroom dance. I lead. She follows. Our connection has reached the point of telepathy as we navigate crowded places. Honey knows when to drop behind my chair to avoid an obstacle and returns to heel without me saying a word. If my chair stops, she sits. If it stops for awhile, she lies down. Honey knows her job and she knows me.

I'm not, "she who must be obeyed," anymore. I'm Honey's partner and dear friend. She's not my servant, a slave to my every command. She helps because she loves to work with me. Working with me gives Honey's life meaning and purpose. You can see it in how she carries herself. Dignified. Proud. Self-assured. Honey is happy and full of life.

The puppy we randomly selected from a litter of mutts in a pet store, turned out to be my perfect service dog. I'm beyond lucky. I'm blessed. When Honey put that pen in my hand as a puppy, she chose this relationship for herself. Honey opened the door; all I did was show her the way through. I'm honored to be partnered with my service dog. My only hope is, she's just as honored to be partnered with me.

Life Music
(for Daddy)

Because I've been to hell and back so many times I've lost count, I named my powerchair, Helen Baaq. Electric purple and black, Helen Baaq is one stylish looking set of wheels. Well, not right now. To tell you the truth, right now Helen Baaq is covered in grayish mud from the Illinois Prairie Path. Helen Baaq often gets muddy when I go out adventuring. Ever since I got my powerchair, I can't stay inside on a nice day. I stayed inside far too many nice days when MG stole the strength in my legs.

I have muscle weakness in my hips that makes walking difficult. On a good day, I can walk around my house. On a bad day, within as few as ten steps I look around for somewhere to sit. Imagine if you could only walk ten steps. What would that do to your life?

Imagine you can't go to work. Or a movie theater. You can't go shopping. Or to a restaurant. Forget about going to church. Your best friend is getting married? Enjoy the video. You're not going to the wedding. There's a new exhibit at the museum. Don't you wish you could go?

Look! The ice cream truck is driving down your street. You didn't want an ice cream, did you?

Gee, doesn't missing out on everything sound like fun? That's why I have a powerchair.

Before I got my chair, I lived on house arrest. No matter how much I wanted to see the lilacs and tulips at our local garden park, I couldn't go. My legs trapped me inside my home, ten steps from the nearest chair. I cried every day the summer of 2004, because I just wanted to take my dog for a walk, but I couldn't do it.

Steve offered to push me in my regular wheelchair through the park and couldn't understand why that made me cry. Independent movement is essential to self-esteem. Sitting in a wheelchair with someone else pushing is not the same thing as choosing where to move, when to move, and how fast to go.

That whole summer I couldn't leave the house by myself. I felt confined and so frustrated I didn't know what to do. Thankfully, I had a neurology appointment in late August. My doctor asked how my summer was going and I broke down.

Understand, I'd seen the same doctor every three months for six years and never cried. No matter how sick I was, I always managed to smile. Stunned, my doctor flung tissues at me and tried to get me to stop crying. I finally calmed down enough to describe how horrible my summer was.

I told him I understood medical science couldn't fix me, but I needed to be able to move. My doctor pulled out a prescription pad and wrote a prescription that changed my life. No, not for a new wonder drug. All it said was, "Indoor and outdoor power wheelchair."

Though it took several months before my chair was delivered, my new chair restored what MG took from me. I remember going for my first long distance powerchair cruise. The new powerchair hummed a friendly electric purr as I went across the street alone. Down the curb cut, zip across the street, up the curb cut and I was off. One block from home. Five blocks. Ten. I was away from home by myself for the first time in five months. I could move. It didn't hurt. It was effortless. I was free.

At a park almost two miles from my home I saw a willow tree. The yellow autumn leaves blew in the wind like confetti. According to the chair manual, my power-chair would go on grass. Should I try? Of course I tried. I rolled my chair under the willow tree and looked up through the leaves at the sky. The willow leaves rained down on me as I spun in joyful circles under the tree. I felt alive and wide awake as I spun around and I didn't care who was watching. Five months of house arrest was over. I was free at last.

My powerchair batteries can go about 15 miles on a charge. The days of struggling to walk Honey around the block are long gone. Now when I take my dog for a walk, it's often ten miles or more. There is nothing I like better than looking at my dog trotting beside my powerchair. I set the speed control as fast as my chair will go and ask Honey, "Wanna go flying?" She always wags her entire body with delight.

I remember the first time I took Honey out with my powerchair. I used a six inch leash to train her to stay beside my chair. Careful not to run over her feet, I took her for the longest walk of her life. She kept looking up at me with an amazed expression on her face. I remember laughing.

Cruising along in Helen Baaq, with Honey at my side, I always feel relieved. Here are two things in my life that help make up for the losses. What dog lover doesn't wish she could bring Fluffy with her everywhere. I get to take my dog everywhere.

Ever ride a go-cart? My powerchair is a lot like a go-cart. Only, I can take it into the mall. Do I feel sorry for myself because I use a powerchair with my best friend at my side? No way! My powerchair is fun to drive and my dog is fun to be with. Every time I zip down our ramp, I'm blissfully happy to be outside and free to move.

One of the best parts about using a wheelchair is buying funky shoes. I don't have to walk in them, so I can buy the most outrageous heels in the store. Better yet, they don't hurt my feet. Last summer, I got myself a pair of black sandals. Open toe with four inch heels, those shoes made me laugh every day. If I wasn't using a wheelchair, I never would have gotten them. I painted my toenails purple to match my chair and wore those ridiculous sandals without fear of falling.

Next summer, I'm looking for more impractical shoes. Someone should invent a line of shoes specifically for wheeler chicks. Eight inch pumps? Bring them my way! When it comes to shoes, the more outrageous the better.

Whenever I think about all of the wonderful advances in medicine, I feel a mixture of excitement and sadness. If a cure for MG came this year, I'd have to give up my service dog and Helen Baaq. I put too much effort into training Honey to retire her and keep her as a pet. Being a pet would break Honey's spirit. So, I'd give Honey away to someone with a disability who needed a trained dog. I'd give my chair away, too. That would be hard to bear. I like my life the way it is. Zooming in my purple powerchair, wearing ridiculous ankle breaking shoes, with a smiling dog trotting faithfully at my side, suits me.

Helen Baaq and Honey enhance my life. Though I never imagined needing a powerchair and a service dog, I'm glad I have them both. They remind me that adapting to change can be fun.

Yes, MG is a disaster. That does not mean my entire life is a disaster. My life works just fine. I can move. I can ask my dog to get me a Pepsi. I can function independently. The music of my life satisfies my soul. It makes me glad to be alive.

A Love Given

In 2004, the MG thief stole my most precious gift. The muscles between my left index finger and thumb atrophied, steadily bending my hand backward into a claw. Of all the losses MG caused, this was the most devastating. Losing strength in my left hand gradually took my cello from me.

For weeks I denied it. I tried to keep practicing, keep teaching lessons, as if nothing was wrong. Then one afternoon, my fingers wouldn't arch properly on the strings. No matter how hard I tried, my fingers angled backward toward my scroll. After seven measures of music, my cello fell silent. I couldn't play anymore.

I did all I could to keep my students from noticing. Instead of playing all of the notes with them, I only played the parts where they were struggling and listened during their lessons. But, when I wasn't teaching, my cello gathered dust on the cello stand. Twenty-six years of music faded from my hands.

I tried to pretend teaching meant more to me than singing sonatas, etudes and concertos. It didn't work. I was devastated. I could adapt to life without walking, without chewing and swallowing normally. I could accept chest surgery and progressive illness. I just didn't know how to accept losing my cello. It hurt like surviving my own death. Everytime I heard cello music, I cried.

Late one December night, I'd just finished crying over my silent cello when I flopped on the couch to watch TV. The sci-fi show I wanted to watch was a rerun, so I flipped through the channels aimlessly. As I made my way around the channels, I heard a man playing guitar.

Only, it wasn't a guitar. It had two necks and fourteen strings. I'd never heard an instrument like it before. Did it sound like a harp? A hammer dulcimer? Whatever it was, the double necked instrument was absolutely beautiful. I set down my remote and just let this music quiet me. The longer he played, the better I felt.

I hoped some kind of announcer would let me know the musician's name so I could get a CD. Before I had a chance to look for a pen and paper, the lovely double necked guitar was joined by a cello.

Rage surged inside me. There on my TV was a woman doing what I loved to do, but couldn't anymore. I almost threw the remote at the screen. I almost started screaming. Instead, I just listened as these two musicians played together, their instruments blending perfectly.

So many emotions ran through me that it felt like stepping inside a tornado. My heart beat fast in my chest, and anger turned my guts inside out. Then the cellist played a glissando and I admired her talent. I sat there

The Dance

thinking, "Wow, she's good." Then I remembered how much I loved playing glissandos. Except, I couldn't play them anymore. It felt like coarse sandpaper scrubbed my insides raw.

The cellist played a note on her highest string. I listened to her vibrato and appreciated her skill. I analyzed the music note by note. I knew where to find each note on my cello and imagined my hands playing. But, I couldn't play anymore.

It's not fair! Why? It's not fair! I snatched the remote to turn it off, but somehow turned up the volume instead. Something about the way the two of them played together captivated me, even though I was still burning up inside.

But, then I saw the woman with the cello smiling a familiar smile. The smile I used to have when I played. The smile of pure cello love. I could tell she played simply because she loved hearing her cello sing, just like I loved hearing my cello sing.

The woman played skillfully and with such tremendous joy, it felt like I was playing again. While I listened, the hurt I felt faded into her cello. Her music made me cry, not because I was jealous, but because I finally felt better. Somehow her music took my pain away.

I didn't even know her name.

The show ended and I learned the name of the duo was Acoustic Eidolon. It was almost two in the morning when I surfed the web and bought a CD and DVD. It felt like an eternity before the package arrived in the mail. Finally I listened, heard that healing music again. I learned the double necked instrument was called a Guitjo. The custom made instrument allows Joe Scott to express himself as a guitarist in a thousand different ways. I also learned the cellist was Hannah Alkire. They're a husband and wife team from a small town in Colorado.

I listened to the CD and watched the DVD several times. Each time I listened, the grief over losing my cello eased. Finally, I wrote an e-mail to Hannah, letting her know I liked her playing very much and that I was a cellist, too. Weeks went by. I'd forgotten I'd ever sent the e-mail when I got a reply.

Hannah told me she enjoyed my e-mail. She said she likes meeting "fellow cellos," and looked forward to meeting me if I could come to an Acoustic Eidolon show.

I read the e-mail twice. Then I looked at my power-chair, and my dusty cello on the cello stand. Realizing I wasn't who Hannah expected to meet, I had a choice to make. Do I reply, let Hannah see me for who I am? Or should I run? I closed my email, turned on my Acoustic Eidolon *Live to Dance* CD and listened to it all the way through.

I listened as Joe played a theme on his Guitjo and then Hannah echoed it on her cello. Sometimes the Guitjo sang while the cello accompanied it. Then they switched. Back and forth they passed the music to one another. It was then I understood why I felt better when Hannah played.

In orchestra, musical themes get passed around from player to player. For example, in the last movement of Beethoven's *Ninth Symphony*, the *Ode to Joy* starts with the cellos and string basses singing by themselves. The rest of the orchestra sits and listens. The second time through the theme, the cellos shift up, the basses accompany the cellos, and a few woodwinds join the party. After that, the entire string section plays while the woodwinds rest. Soon, the brass section, woodwinds, and percussion add their voices to the strings and the whole orchestra plays together.

When the entire orchestra plays the *Ode to Joy*, we're having a collective Beethoven love festival on stage. It sounds incredible. Playing it is life changing. Of all the music I've ever played in orchestra, I loved playing Beethoven the best. Makes my heart beat fast just thinking about it.

In orchestra, every musician knows sometimes you rest and listen to the music. Or, you play harmony parts, accompanying someone else gently. Then you get the melody back and sing out with your soul. In orchestra, I've always known that when the cello section rests, the music didn't die. It merely changed hands.

While listening to Hannah play her cello, I understood why I felt better. The music inside me didn't die. It just changed hands. As long as Hannah could play what my heart wanted to say, the music inside me would go on.

Somehow, I had to let her know. So, I took a risk and told this stranger the truth about me. I e-mailed Hannah and let her know I was very sick and couldn't play my cello anymore. I told her every other cellist made me jealous. Listening to cello music felt like teasing on the playground, "Ha ha, listen to what I can do. Don't you wish you could do it, too?" In my e-mail, I wrote that Hannah's playing didn't feel like teasing.

Then I offered Hannah my baton, as if we were running a relay race. I told her to take my love for the cello, because I couldn't play anymore. I let her know I was trusting her to play what was stuck inside my soul, because she'd already done it. I knew as long as she had my baton, the music inside me would be safe in her hands.

I took a deep breath, and clicked send.

The next day, Hannah e-mailed me back, graciously accepting my baton. Hannah wrote many things that comfort me to this day. But, then she did something that I did not expect. Just like I took a risk and decided to let her in, Hannah took a risk and decided to let me in.

She wrote me about her battle with non-Hodgkin's lymphoma. Through my tears, I read Hannah's e-mail. Here was a stranger who knew what it felt like to fight for her life. She took cancer classes at The University of Catastrophe, just like me. Hannah fought hard for her life, and for her cello, and won them both.

As I read her encouraging words, a thought ran through my mind. Maybe I've given up on my cello too easily. Perhaps I needed to fight for my cello just as hard as I fought for my life.

A Love Returned

(For Hannah, who still has my baton)

I took my dusty cello off the stand and sat down in the music room. Just like always, after a few measures of playing, my left hand collapsed. Only, instead of breaking down in tears, I finally analyzed what was wrong. Because of the atrophy in my left thumb, my hand bent at the wrong angle. What if I arched my hand differently? Concentrating on keeping my hand balanced, I pressed on. That afternoon, I started reinventing how to play the cello. It didn't sound like it used to, but I was playing again.

Ecstatic, I returned to my computer and e-mailed my new friend about my discoveries. Hannah e-mailed me back, celebrating my victories.

Week by week, I kept experimenting. I tried using a violin bow, because I kept dropping my cello bow. Violin bows are lighter than cello bows, so that helped. I tried putting my left hand in different places on the cello neck. I kept trying, teaching myself how to play the cello again. Meanwhile, Hannah cheered me on.

169

Via e-mail, we discovered we have a lot in common beyond playing the cello. We're both wives and mothers. We both have a sense of wonder and are in love with life. How about this? We even went to the same cello camp as kids, just a few years apart! Our common experiences, both good and bad, are absolutely uncanny. Hannah and I discovered we're two halves of the same walnut and quickly became dear friends. We both looked forward to Acoustic Eidolon's November concert in the Chicago area when we could finally meet.

Hannah and I exchanged emails for two months when Acoustic Eidolon's east coast tour wrapped. That weekend, Hannah had a concert in Champaign Illinois and after some thought, Hannah realized she was going to be only three hours south of my house. OK, remember the safety rules about people you meet online? Well, some rules are made to be broken.

On a Wednesday in May 2005, Hannah wheeled her cello case up my wheelchair ramp into my house. At first, Hannah and I were a bit awkward. Was I who Hannah thought I was? Was Hannah who I thought she was? Was meeting a good idea or not? That didn't last, and soon we were laughing and goofing around.

We sat down with our cellos in my music room. Now, obviously, I was too intimidated to play. So, Hannah said, "Hey, do you know how to make your cello moo?"

"Excuse me?" I said, eyes wide.

"Moo. You know, like a cow." Hannah demonstrated the most ridiculous sound on her cello.

I burst out laughing, and quickly got over being scared. We traded cellos and admired each other's voices.

Though the notes are the same, all cellos feel and sound different. Her cello, Gypsy Girl, has a joyful laughing brilliance in her tone that is so totally Hannah it made me laugh to play her.

Hannah played my cello, Sir. Barclay, and after a few notes exclaimed, "He's so sweet!" He is. My cello has a richness and a sweet gentle tone that matches me and my personality perfectly.

We played cellos until my hands got too tired. Then we went for a long walk. Well, Hannah walked. I power-chair hiked. I even let Hannah go for a dizzying spin in my powerchair. During that walk we talked for hours.

That afternoon wasn't like being with a new friend. It wasn't like being with an old friend. It was like spending time with a part of myself that was always missing, and finally found. I remember being startled the planets didn't spin out of axis.

Later that afternoon, we played cellos in Lilacia Park, surrounded by lilacs and tulips. For 26 years, I was a classical cellist. As a kid, I was taught to play the notes on the paper and play them correctly. It never occurred to me to seriously venture outside of the box. The only thing I played other than classical music was bluegrass.

I love bluegrass. Ten years ago I got myself a fiddle and taught myself to play. Now, I have no problem telling you, I am a truly horrible fiddle player. So, I learn bluegrass tunes on my fiddle just long enough to transfer them to my cello. Then I can really wail! But, I never considered fiddle tunes on a cello anything more than a curiosity. The cello is a classical instrument. That's what I was taught. That's what I knew.

Sitting on a park bench, Hannah played everything except classical music on her cello: folk music, bits of flamenco, tunes she made up on the fly, even rock. I sat there listening and kept asking, "Wait! How are you doing that?" Hannah slowed it down, showed me how she played the impossible. Of course, I started laughing. "That's nuts! I can't do that."

"Yes, you can. See, it's like this. And then you do this."

I tried, failed, tried again, then figured out what Hannah was doing. "I think I got it!"

"See, I told you, you could do it!"

Happy that I learned something new, I launched into a fiddle tune, playing my cello hoedown style. I was playing the double shuffle in *Bile Them Cabbage Down* when Hannah abruptly stopped playing.

"Wait!" she said, "How are you doing that?"

This time I slowed down, showed Hannah how I was playing the shuffle and waited until she got it. In the park, we had a wonderful time playing cellos and trading styles of music. Too soon it was time for her to go back to Champaign. It was a day neither of us will ever forget.

After Hannah left, I kept experimenting with my cello. The muscle weakness in my hands makes it impossible for me to play classical music. But, it doesn't make it impossible for me to play. Inspired by the afternoon with my friend, I began composing. At first, I felt like I was breaking rules. Am I allowed to compose music? Me? After all, even when I improvised, I riffed off someone else's tune. Could I play music I made up myself? To my delight, not only could I compose, but through composing I rediscovered my love for the cello.

Because of MG, I physically cannot play some notes. My left hand won't move with enough dexterity anymore. Composing lets me get around that limitation. I compose what I can play, and I find a level of satisfaction and joy in playing my cello that I've never known before. I thought my cello was silenced forever. Instead, because of Hannah, Sir. Barclay was given back to me more mine than ever before.

I've always thought of the cello as my voice, a way I can express the life inside me that goes beyond words. Playing classical music taught me how to play tenderly, or harshly, and I learned to express the full range of emotions through my cello. But, when I composed music, I finally took my cello's voice and made it my own.

For the first time, I felt like my cello completely belonged to me. Not to Bach or Beethoven's dreams for my cello, but my own. Composing lets me sing out of myself, singing of the life within me.

With Hannah's encouragement, I returned to the studio as a solo artist. Headphones on, cello in front of a microphone, I recorded my own compositions and loved every moment. Instead of just running ahead with my baton, Hannah helped me find my cello again, and not only though helping me learn to compose. In August 2005, it was clear my MG progressed far enough to seriously threaten my life. To survive, I needed to start IV chemotherapy, even though I was petrified.

Having fought cancer, Hannah knew what I was walking into and held a light for me. Hannah talked me through losing my hair and eyebrows. She helped me handle the side effects from the anti-nausea drugs, and gave me comfort and strength when I was terrified.

At my first oncology appointment, I handed my new doctor my cello bow. I told her, I didn't need to be able to see, or eat, or walk. All I needed was to be able to play the cello again. My doctor told me she would try.

Chemotherapy saved my life. It saved my cello as well. Within a few cycles, I noticed the atrophy in my hand reversing. Muscle grew back into the space between my index finger and thumb. Muscle grew in my right shoulder so I could hold my cello bow again. Before chemotherapy, I could play the cello in brief 15 minute bursts. Now Sir. Barclay and I can sing for hours. Just like my friend Hannah, I have my life, and my cello both, and I am amazed.

Obviously, Hannah and I e-mail and talk on the phone as often as we can. She invited me to visit her in Colorado and we had a blast together. We'll find a way to visit one another sometime soon.

I'm looking forward to playing cello with Hannah again, listening to her play notes I swear aren't on my cello and howling with laughter when she plays Sir. Barclay and proves me wrong. But, most of all, I'm looking forward to all the wonderful things life has in store for my dear friend Hannah and me.

Weaving Part II

E ver wonder how people in the ancient world heard about the news? I mean, they couldn't stroll up to an internet café and go online, or even pick up a newspaper. And what did they do for entertainment without TV, radio, movies and books? Who told the people of distant battles, or how the harvest was going in the north? Who told them about a new road being built in the south? Who taught everyone about the world beyond their homes?

Since the stone age, people have gathered together and listened to storytellers. In our modern world, we gather around the blue glow of TV sets instead of flickering fires. But, we're still doing what our ancestors did when we watch stories on TV. People need stories. Stories are how we connect with each other.

"Remember the time when we were in the car and the fog..."

"The funniest thing happened to me on the way home from the train. I was walking past this fire hydrant when..."

"My scar? Oh, I got that when I was seven. See, I was riding my bike across…"

We learn about the world through stories. For centuries, the professional storyteller was the keeper of myth, legend, and also a truth teller. For many people, their only source of accurate information was from the traveling bard. No wonder the bard was so highly regarded.

> Bards are honored and respected throughout the world, for the muse teaches them their songs and loves them.
>
> Homer, *The Odyssey*
> Greek Poet (800 BC - 700 BC)

The idea of a traveling bard captivated me when I was a child. In fifth grade, I was in a huge Junior Girl Scout troop. Almost all of the girls in my school's fifth grade classes were in this troop. I remember having a wonderful time with all of my friends. I also remember the first time I told a story around a campfire.

After we ate our obligatory burnt hot dogs, sandy potato chips, and gobbled down s'mores, the firelight flickered, and I told a scary story for all of the girls. I made the story up as I went along, and I could see the girls leaning forward on their logs. They jumped in fright and gasped. Then they cheered at the end. After I finished my story one of the leaders talked to me about it. She couldn't believe I made it up, but I did. Right then and there, I decided I wanted to be a storyteller when I grew up. Even better, I wanted to be a storyteller who played music. I wanted to be a bard.

Admitting I wanted to be a bard wasn't something I told anyone. It was the 1980's not the 1380's! Frankly, the idea just sounded too ridiculous to voice. So, I studied music and language arts separately and gave up on the idea of bringing them together. Still, deep inside, I wanted to be a bard. I felt like I was born in the wrong century.

Then I ended up at The University of Catastrophe. All of my dreams and desires were gobbled up faster than the Girl Scouts ate s'mores. After I was diagnosed with thymoma positive MG, I wanted to do one thing: survive. That was my mission and focus for many years. I didn't have time to chase childhood dreams.

I got through freshman year at The University of Catastrophe holding on with white knuckles and screaming. Sophomore year, I looked inward and tried to figure out how to find inner peace. Junior year, I looked outward at the world, raging at how I was typecast in a role I never auditioned for or wanted. Senior year, I learned to laugh at the world's reactions to my disability, and honor my own strengths. I learned to wear the scarlet *D* for *Disability* with dignity and grace.

The University of Catastrophe doesn't always end senior year, though. Without my consent, I was enrolled in graduate school. Right now I have a Master of Medical Mayhem. I'm still in graduate school, working toward my Doctorate in Doctor's Appointments. I've taken graduate seminars like *Faith: You Can Lose It. Faith II: You Can Find It. Trees, Flowers, Birds and Mountains: You Can Appreciate*

Them. Just like in my undergrad years, I've learned a lot in graduate school. Right now I'm taking, *Dreams: You Can Chase Them*. And I'm looking forward to starting *Dreams II: You Can Catch Them.*

As soon as I started taking *Dreams: You Can Chase Them*, part of my spirit I thought had died woke up and started to burn. The class began over a glass of wine at Hannah's dining room table. Hannah was talking about working on stage with Acoustic Eidolon. I nibbled my cheese, sipped my wine, and asked questions.

Then Hannah suggested I could give a performance, sharing what I've learned about life, and play my cello for people. She even told me that my service dog could be in the show.

I choked on my wine! Excuse me? Talking to a group of people? Had she lost her mind? Doesn't Hannah realize I took a speech class in junior high and I was horrible at public speaking? I remember puking in a trash can before my speech. I wisely avoided public speaking ever since. That's when I knew Hannah had too much wine, and was mistaking me for someone else.

There is an Irish proverb: "A friend's eye is a good mirror." Sometimes, our friends see things in us that we don't see in ourselves. Somehow over that glass of wine, Hannah looked into my eyes and saw a silent bard.

While I was flying home from Colorado, I scribbled in my journal about talking to people and playing music for them. I pictured myself weaving between storytelling and music, sharing what I've learned. What would I say? Would anyone listen?

I wrote in my journal for months, trying to figure out how to put together a performance. I practiced speaking to an imaginary audience. I composed music to fit between the stories. On the phone, Hannah suggested I give my show a name. Several weeks later, I named my performance *Weaving: an Inspirational Journey*.

Rev. Ed Searl, the minister at my childhood church, offered me the opportunity to debut my show on a Sunday morning in July 2006. That morning, I did exactly what I practiced. I spoke about my life's journey. Waking up blind and in agony, and 16 doctors being unable to diagnose what was wrong. Finding out I had myasthenia gravis and getting my eyesight back. I talked about the 4x3x2 centimeter tumor growing in my chest and surviving the surgery from hell.

After playing my cello, I talked about living in a sandcastle, and blending illness into my life like stirring lemon into tea. Then I shifted directions, and talked about disability and adaptive equipment. I talked about the word inspiring and what it means to inspire: giving life, breath, spirit, to someone. It's not inspiring to go shopping while seated in a wheelchair.

I told them about Honey and showed everyone what she can do to help me. Pretending I was in the grocery store, I dropped a can of soup, a bag of chips, a pen, a credit card and a dime. Honey retrieved them all for me, just like she always does. But, then I told them about what Honey can't do. She can't help me with the questions that eat at my soul. I spoke of suicide and the path to choose life. Then I summarized the whole journey in a song called *Weaving*.

Between each segment, I played my cello and sang songs from my spirit. After talking about losing my sight and getting it back again, I played *Orange on Blue*, a song about seeing a maple tree, dressed for autumn, stretched out against a clear Illinois blue sky. Back and forth, I talked and played music. I shared truth and struggles, tears and laughter.

In that moment, I became the bard I always secretly dreamed I could be. Sometimes, if you chase a dream you just might catch it. It's easy to give up on dreams. They seem like fragile things because they burst like balloons when someone throws darts at them. Sometimes we fling darts at our own dreams. I've learned something about dreams, though: failure hurts less than not trying at all.

When I first started performing *Weaving: an Inspirational Journey*, I was scared of making a mistake on stage. I'm all alone out there. If someone plays a honking horrible note on the cello, I can't pretend it was the other guy. There's a cello joke that goes like this:

"How do you get a cellist to play loud?"

"Mark the music, 'Quiet, but very expressive.'"

"How do you get a cellist to play soft?"

"Mark the music, 'Solo. '"

I wasn't used to playing solo cello. I felt such stage fright it was hard to play. Then I thought of two words that made my stage fright go away: stage version. That wasn't a mistake, it was just the stage version, so keep right on going. Besides, mistakes are part of every journey.

Even better, sometimes what was humiliating a few weeks ago can become hilarious.

So if you dream of starting a business, I encourage you to start one. If you always wanted to travel, plan a trip and go. I encourage you to reach for your dreams, and do the work to make them come true. I've learned that no one else is gonna do it for you. I've also learned life is too short to ignore your dreams. Be bold. Take one step toward your dream. I'm sure glad I did.

Wild Ride

In January 2006, I asked my neurologist if I was well enough to get my driver's license. More than a few doctors have looked into my eyes and said, "Um, you don't drive, do you, Marie?" So, I thought he would say no, too.

I was feeling stronger than I had in many years, and I didn't see double anymore. I thought my neurologist would balk, but instead he told me to go right ahead and get my driver's license. Yay! Except for one minor little problem.

I didn't know how to drive.

Steve drove me home from my neurology appointment and I told him that my doctor said I could get my driver's license. My husband smiled at me. "Cool. Drive me home."

Since I was looking out the window on Illinois Rt. 83 at the time, with traffic zipping along at 65 miles an hour, my eyes widened. "What? Are you insane? I can't!"

Steve laughed. "No problem. It's not rocket science. I'll teach you how to drive."

As soon as I got home, I studied the rules of the road. Then the next day I got a learner's permit at the DMV. I remember looking at the permit and wondering if I was in over my head. On the way home from the DMV, Steve drove us to a park. He pulled into the empty parking lot and stopped the car. Just like any beginner, I climbed into the driver's seat and buckled my seatbelt. That's when I discovered something crucial.

I didn't know how to start a car.

Steve told me how to start the car, and how to put it in drive. "OK, put your foot on the gas and give it a little squeeze."

As soon as the car rolled forward, I stamped on the brake. Hard! Steve's still complaining about whiplash. Just the idea of making a car move scared me to death. I took some deep breaths and then put my foot on the gas again. This time we rolled forward at five miles an hour in the empty lot. I felt like I was speeding.

I made a wide left turn and had a sinking feeling I'd never get the hang of driving a car. But, Steve kept coaching me and I went around and around the parking lot, making wide left turns. Then, Steve suggested I should try going the other way and make right turns.

This felt even worse! I just couldn't get the hang of making a right turn. The car seemed to have a mind of its own. I was about to ask Steve a question when another car came into the lot. I hit the brakes and freaked out. Steve, who was trying not to laugh, traded places with me and drove us home. But, I drove! I was elated. Steve took me to the same parking lot every day to practice. I still made ridiculously wide turns.

Early the next Sunday, Steve drove us to an empty industrial park. Real streets, with stop signs and everything, but not a car in sight. Perfect. I wasn't ready to share the road. I wasn't ready to drive more than ten miles an hour! That Sunday, I drove around and around past empty factories, gaining confidence with every turn.

Now, I'd only been driving for a week when I made a wrong turn out of the industrial park. I suddenly found myself on a six lane busy highway with cars flying past.

Before I had a chance to panic, Steve calmly said, "Put your foot on the gas and ease up to the speed of the other cars."

I did that, while holding the steering wheel in a death grip. "What do I do? What do I do?"

Still sounding calm, Steve said, "Flip on your turn signal, slow down, and turn right."

I barely knew how to make a right turn, or slow down, but I flicked the turn signal, squeezed the brake, and turned right. We ended up in an empty parking lot. I remember putting the car in park and making a fast exit for the safety of the passenger seat. Meanwhile, Steve cheered, telling me what a great job I did. I remember shaking. A lot.

Week by week, my confidence grew. Steve took me on Sunday morning adventures, teaching me different skills. Learning to drive in heavy traffic took a while for me, but I did it. I also learned all of the maneuvers to pass the test at the DMV.

Because of the cognitive changes from the chemotherapy, learning to back up our car was tough. I just couldn't figure out how to think in reverse. Poor Steve tried so hard to teach me. He kept telling me, "Which way do you want your butt to go?" But, parts of my brain software are corrupted. The words *left* and *right* have lost some of their meaning. But, I figured out a way around it.

Before I put the car in reverse, I decide which way I need to turn the wheel. I look for an object to either the left or the right of the car, like a tree or a building. So I think, "I want to turn the wheel toward the tree," before I back up. Then I put the car in reverse, turn the wheel toward the tree, and safely back up the car.

Backing up may never be on automatic pilot for me, and that's OK. Learning to drive taught me that it's all right to take an extra few seconds to figure things out. Life is not a game show and there isn't a buzzer that sounds if you take things slower.

I really found that out when I went for my driver's license test. At the DMV, I got in the car by myself for the first time. It was weird driving without Steve beside me, even if I was just driving around a parking lot. Then a nice older gentleman from the DMV sat beside me with his little clipboard.

I drove him around town, making sure not to speed. I remembered to signal and stop just the way Steve taught me. Then the DMV guy told me to drive to the park, so I did. That's when things got a little weird.

The man told me to back around a corner in the parking lot. I did that, carefully backing around a concrete island. Then he told me to leave the park, and turn right. So, I drove into the driveway and stopped. On my left, two cars were coming, so I patiently waited for them to pass, before making my right turn. I even remembered to flick on my turn signal.

While I was waiting, an SUV slightly larger than a Sherman tank drove up behind me in the park. He got within a few inches of my bumper and laid on the horn. I didn't want to cut off the other two cars, so I waited for them, and then made my right turn.

Mr. Road Rage turned behind me, honking his horn and waving at me with his middle finger. The speed limit is 25 on that street, so I drove 25 miles an hour, ignoring the insane driver behind me. What else was I supposed to do? Speed? I had the DMV officer in my car!

At a stop sign, I came to a complete stop, paused to a count of three, looked both ways for imaginary traffic, and then continued on my way. The audacity of actually coming to a complete stop at a stop sign unhinged Mr. Road Rage. He got so close, I thought he was gonna shove my car across the street.

After the stop sign, I sped up to, you guessed it, 25 miles an hour, calmly ignoring the lunatic behind me. The DMV guy grumbled about the jerk, but I just kept pretending Mr. Road Rage wasn't there, and followed the rules of the road.

Honk! Honk! No matter what I did, the crazy SUV driver just wouldn't stop tailgating me, or screaming obscenities. And there I was taking my first driver's test!

At a stop light, Mr. Road Rage made a wild right turn on red, cutting off other drivers, and nearly causing an accident. I watched him go, grateful he wasn't behind me anymore. The DMV guy told me he was impressed by how calmly I handled Mr. Road Rage.

That was the last part of my driving test, so I drove the DMV guy back to the parking lot. As I was pulling into a parking space, there was a red pole right in front of my car. The man joked, "Don't hit the pole!"

"I'm not gonna hit the pole!" I said, laughing. I pulled up within inches of the pole and put the car in park.

So, I passed my driver's license test on my first try. As I was leaving the DMV with Steve, the guy who gave me my behind the wheel test was talking to his coworkers about Mr. Road Rage. All of them waved to me and smiled. Looking at them, I got the feeling I could have screwed up half of the behind the wheel test and still passed, just because Mr. Road Rage didn't rattle my cage.

I still don't let maniac drivers bother me, although I do get annoyed when people don't signal. Or fly past me on the right, then cut me off only to arrive at a stoplight a whole second ahead of me. Or when I try to change lanes and the car next to me matches my speed to block me. Drives me nuts!

But, the true lunatics like Mr. Road Rage... I just get out of their way, even if it means making a right turn off the road. Whenever I see a total lunatic, I assume the driver is either on drugs, armed, or both. I've studied enough at The University of Catastrophe. I don't need to attend *Surviving a Gunshot*. Or *Handcuffs: One Size Fits All*.

That night, I took my first solo journey. I thought I was going to go on a nice simple cruise through the neighborhood. That's not what happened. I was heading west on a familiar street and I was supposed to make a left turn and head for home. But, I missed the left turn. No matter. I figured I'd make a right turn, go around the block, and end up right back where I started.

Nope. I ended up on a winding street and got lost. I tried to circle back to where I started, but I was in a maze of winding streets and cul-de-sacs. Somehow, I ended up miles north of my house, on Lake Street, which is a busy road. Lake Street was under construction and the lanes were barely wide enough for a bicycle. Sawhorses blinked orange in a maze of seemingly random lane changes.

I'd never driven in a construction zone.

"Remember what Steve taught you and just stay in your lane." I repeated this in a mantra as I drove 45 miles an hour behind semi-trucks and around car swallowing gaps in the road. I looked for familiar road signs, but they'd all evaporated.

Then I decided maybe a business would give me a clue where I was. There was a Home Depot, a Wal-Mart, a Taco Bell, and a McDonald's, and… Great! Am I in Illinois? Kansas? How did I end up in Rhode Island? On my first day with my shiny new driver's license, I was hopelessly lost. Driving 45 miles an hour. In the dark. In heavy traffic. In a construction zone!

Finally, I found a street I recognized. I made a right turn and started driving toward home. Thank God. Except, nothing looked familiar. I knew I was pretty far north of my house so I kept driving, hoping I'd see something I recognized. After about ten minutes, it dawned on me – I was on the right road, but driving in the wrong direction! I found a place to turn around, and ended up back on the familiar road, and headed toward home.

Boy, was I glad to pull into my driveway and turn off the car. Baptism by fire? No, that was baptism by construction! I did it. But, I'll admit, as soon as I got through the front door I poured myself a stiff one. I needed it after that.

Because he loves me, and because I'm directionally challenged, Steve just bought me a TomTom GPS unit for my car. So, now I have a nifty little gadget that knows exactly where I am, even if I don't have a clue. A few days ago, I got lost on purpose just to test my new gadget.

In a parking lot, I pushed a few buttons on my TomTom. Like magic, satellites figured out my exact location on the globe and sent that information to my GPS unit. Poof! My gizmo showed me a map of where I was and a friendly electronic voice told me how to get home. "Turn left. Then take the second right."

Yay! I made it home stress free. My TomTom didn't even route me through a construction zone. I think I'm in love! Thanks, Steve!

Now I understand why people fall in love with their cars. There's incredible freedom in driving. Cruising around with the windows down, iPod playing my favorite songs, has got to be one of life's greatest pleasures. I used to read Braille and walk with a white cane. Now, I can drive a car. Can you believe it? Talk about a wild ride!

Gray? No Way!

January 8, 2007, I completed my 23rd cycle of IV chemotherapy. After 18 months of continuous chemo, the side effects overwhelmed me. Like a broad spectrum insecticide, the chemotherapy killed cells throughout my body. Hair loss I could deal with. The cognitive changes I couldn't handle anymore.

I vividly remember trying to put groceries away and holding a bag of frozen peas. I knew it was a bag of peas. I knew peas were green, round, and tasted good with butter and salt. I just couldn't remember if frozen peas belonged in the freezer or the cupboard. So, I held them, feeling the coldness on my skin. But, even the cold sensation wasn't enough to trigger what to do with the frozen peas.

Tears filled my eyes because I understood that I should *know* what to do with the peas. I've been putting groceries away since I was five. I just couldn't connect the dots. Month after month of chemotherapy marinated my brain. I felt like a superfund site. While I stood in the kitchen holding that bag of peas, I felt hopeless and stupid.

As usual, when I couldn't make a simple decision, I started crying like a little kid.

I completely understand why toddlers meltdown when they can't find their favorite toy bunny. The last time they remember seeing the bunny, it was on the table next to their bed. But, it's not there, so the kid loses it.

Frustrated parents ask, "Did you look under your bed? Did you look in your toy box?" To an adult, those seem like such obvious next steps.

But, it takes critical thinking skills to first get past the surprise of, "Oh no, where's my fuzzy bunny?" Followed by a logical leap, "Wait, I bet I left it on the sofa." Little ones hit the surprise, but they don't have the thinking skills to figure out the next step to solve the problem, so they cry.

Standing in the kitchen, holding a now warm bag of peas, I lost it sobbing. *Where do these go? I should know, but I can't remember. Peas. They're peas. They're in a bag. Some peas go in the freezer. But some peas go in the cupboard. Do cans go in the cupboard or do bags? I can't remember. Why can't I remember. I should know this.*

Evelyn heard me crying and came running. "What's wrong?"

I told her, "I don't know where these go. Do they go in the... the..." I searched in vain for the word *freezer*, but it was deleted from my memory. "That big box that keeps food cold. Or the cupboard?"

My 16-year-old daughter took the peas and quietly put them in the freezer. Then she gave me a hug and repeatedly whispered, "I love you, Mom," while I cried on her shoulder. Then Evelyn put the rest of the groceries away.

I lost myself in a toxic chemical brain bath. I had word recall problems. Confusion. Memory lapses. I got lost a few blocks from home and couldn't remember how to get back. I couldn't remember how to write a check. The potato button on the microwave confused me when I was trying to make cream of potato soup. Do I push the potato button to cook potato soup?

Month after month, I lost more and more of my mind. At 37, this was terrifying! What would I be like in six months? Or a year? I could handle losing the use of my body, but what about my mind?

In February 2007, I cried during my chemotherapy appointment. A 24th cycle of chemotherapy was more than I could bear. My oncologist told me that if I was fighting cancer, I'd have gotten to skip a cycle months ago. But, my myasthenia gravis wouldn't allow a break. My doctor explained to me that if 18 months of non-stop IV treatment didn't make my MG go into remission, 18 more months would do it, either.

My doctor dried my tears. She wrote me a prescription for a different chemotherapy drug. It was less toxic. They were pills I could take at home once a week. Then my doctor looked at me and laughed, "Oh, by the way, you'll be able to grow back your hair!"

Wait, did she say I could grow back my hair? My own hair? I remember almost bouncing out of the office! That night I took the chemotherapy pills. I also barfed, which sucked. I've since learned to take anti-nausea drugs, then the chemo pills, and then more anti-nausea drugs. But, that night I didn't know any better, so I barfed.

The next day, I felt... fine. Well, fine for me. That was so weird. No steroids making me feel jumpy. No anti-nausea drugs making me feel sleepy and foggy. I could move and play my cello the day after chemo. Wow! I didn't get a needle stick in my port, or have to spend hours in the treatment room. No chemo cave. Such a deal! I felt like I was cheating.

A few weeks later, I had fuzz growing on my head. I looked in the mirror and smiled. Hooray! I've got hair. My eyelashes slowly grew back in and stopped itching. I still haven't grown back my eyebrows all the way, but I don't care. They used to be too bushy, anyway.

The new chemotherapy suppresses my appetite, so I'm steadily losing weight. After months of steroids making me steadily gain weight, I'm thrilled. I mean, weight loss as a side effect? Oh how horrifying! If I get down to a size zero, I'll worry about it. Until then, I'm watching the numbers on the scale go down, down, down and that rocks.

Gradually, I noticed the brain fog lifting. That was such a relief. I can go shopping and not feel like crying because I can't find the right brand of tea. I can put frozen peas away and not worry that I'll get confused anymore.

I still have some cognitive problems, but they're mild now. My mind sometimes stalls like a manual transmission car if you let out the clutch too fast. But, I can get my mind in gear a whole lot quicker than before. I'm learning to connect the dots again, and that makes me happy.

Did I mention I have hair? I do. I have enough hair to brush. I have enough hair to pull. I can twist my fingers in my bangs and loop a spiral curl. My hair grew back in curly, but not as curly as before. And... gray! Oh no!

OK, not exactly gray. It grew in dark brown with gray. When my hair first grew back, the tips were almost all gray, and that alarmed me. As it grew longer, some of the gray hairs darkened, but not enough. Good grief! I'm not even 40 yet! I'm not supposed to have this much gray hair.

Did you know that The University of Catastrophe has a beauty school? I took a class called *Your Head: Your Personal Palette*. Just last week, I went to Walgreen's to buy my first bottle of hair color.

I looked at the shades to choose from. Platinum blonde? Copper red? Black? Green? As I looked at all of my choices, I didn't feel confusion edging into my mind. Just a few months ago so many choices would have overloaded the circuit board. But, not anymore. I almost did a powerchair whirl in excitement, but I contained myself. Instead I selected a box that promised me dark auburn hair.

That night I put on plastic gloves and covered my hair in smelly goop. Did I mind the smell? Heck no! I had hair! Twenty-five minutes and a long rinse later, I had dark auburn hair. And there wasn't a single gray strand mocking me in the mirror. *Aging Gracefully Is Optional* was a really fun class. I'll take it again in a few weeks.

Next year, I'll have my braid back. Growing my hair long is important to me. Next time I braid my hair I'll close the door on the grueling IV chemo adventure. It was worth the journey, but I'm glad I'm on a different road. This road is a whole lot easier.

At The University of Catastrophe, I studied *Hair: You Can Lose It. Your Brain: It Can Be Pickled. Steroids and You: Look! Your Scale Can Go Higher.* Those classes all sucked.

Here in graduate school, I'm taking *Hair: You Can Grow it. Your Brain: It Can Recover. Weight: You Can Lose it. The Car: You Can Make It Zoom. Your Cello: You Can Play It. The Stage: Welcome Home.* And best of all, I'm taking *The Future: You Can Enjoy It.* No wonder I wake up and feel like dancing.

For Life
(for Steve)

Here it is, Monday night again. I still hate Mondays, even during football season. This evening, I took some anti-nausea drugs and my chemotherapy pills. So here I am, three hours after swallowing a handful of tablets and my guts are churning like I'm about to barf. Imagine having the stomach flu every Monday night. It's tough. I'm tougher.

If I stop chemotherapy, my MG will overwhelm me. My hands will atrophy and I won't be able to play my cello. I won't be able to drive anymore. I'll end up right back where I started, struggling to breathe, and unable to chew and swallow. If I stop taking chemotherapy, I'll die. How I ended up in this predicament, I don't know.

On April 14, 1997, I was an ordinary 27-year-old wife and mother. Now, I've had more needle sticks than a pincushion, and swallowed enough pills to stock my neighborhood drug store. Unless a new drug, or treatment comes along, I'll be taking chemotherapy in some form or another for the rest of my life. I could view this as a life sentence. But, I don't. I'm taking chemotherapy *for* life.

I'm taking chemotherapy because I want to see my daughter graduate from high school. I want to see Evelyn graduate from college. Get a job. Get married. I want to hug my son-in-law. See my daughter become a mother. I want to hold my first grandchild in my arms.

I want to visit my daughter's home and see how Evelyn decorates it. She has a flair for decorating. I want to see what she does with her home and life.

I want to see the sunset over Lake Michigan from Sleeping Bear Dunes in 2008. Feel the heat of the sand on my fingers. Feel the lake cool my toes. I want to toss rocks in the lake and hear them splash. I want to find pieces of green glass polished by tumbling in Lake Michigan. I want to hold them in my hand and wonder how long they've been in the lake. Did a glass bottle break in 1947 in Chicago and the shattered pieces drift to the Michigan shore? I want to touch the polished glass. I want to wonder.

I want to watch a thunderstorm, see lightning flash in the sky and hear thunder roll. Sitting on the porch watching the wind in the trees, I want to feel the mist of rain on my skin, and the way my heart jumps at every crash of thunder. I want to see the next storm. And the one after that.

What if an aurora borealis lights up the sky in 2011? I want to look up and see the colors swirl and dance. I want to see the stars in the Rocky Mountains again. See Cassiopeia so close I could touch it. Then I want to shut my eyes and listen to the silence of the mountains, aware of the stillness, and my own breathing. I want to live to see the first snow of 2012. The first delicate purple crocus blossom of 2016. I want to live to see it all.

I'm taking chemotherapy so I can pay my electric bill, and then do the laundry with Honey's help. Drive around town running errands. Go grocery shopping with my dog. Make pasta salad while Steve cooks chicken on the barbeque grill. Sitting outside sipping wine, watching fireflies light up our backyard, reveling in the ordinary the summer of 2010, is worth fighting for.

I want to be here to help my husband fix a flat tire on a Tuesday. Install a new toilet. Clean up another broken mug. Wake up to the sound of a cat puking on the bed and panic. Laugh at a movie. Decorate the Christmas tree with my family.

I want to visit London with Steve and laugh because he won't have jet lag. His work schedule has him on London time already. I need to be here for that.

There are places I need to see. Foods I need to try. New songs hiding on my cello waiting for my fingers to find them. There is recording I need to do. Concerts I need to perform. I need so much to be alive.

I'm taking chemotherapy so I can get in a horrible fight with Steve and then make up and rebuild our marriage. So I can watch the news and cry. So I can attend a funeral for someone I loved and grieve. So I can go to a wedding and laugh as the bride throws her bouquet.

Chemotherapy is for getting the mail in cold November drizzle, tossing junk mail in the fireplace, and watching the flames consume the paper to ash. For getting a cold and sneezing. It's for sitting up with Evelyn when she's sick and holding her in my arms. It's so I can be here to console my daughter when she breaks up with her boyfriend. So I can look at the clock and worry that Evelyn isn't home yet, and feel relieved when she walks into the house safe and sound.

It's for visiting Hannah in Colorado and playing cellos together and laughing. For crying in the airport when it's time to go home. For hugging Steve and Evelyn in Chicago and being glad to see them again. It's for greeting the joyful dogs when I get home.

I'm taking chemotherapy so I can watch the birds build nests in our maple tree. Watch the robins fly to and from the tree, and listen to the baby birds chirping when their parents arrive. I want to see the daffodils in my garden bloom in the spring. And the next spring. And the next. I want to visit the garden park and watch the tulips sway in the breeze. Then play my cello for the flowers, and the people in the park, and for the sky.

I'm taking chemotherapy so I can live. For travel. And homecomings. For grief. And laughter. For all of the beautiful things to see in this world. For mundane afternoons vacuuming dog hair off the rug. For being depressed. And elated. For singing. For dancing. For life.

About The Author

Marie Culbert Smith grew up in LaGrange, Illinois. She studied music and writing at The Interlochen Arts Academy in Interlochen, Michigan. She was also a member of the Chicago Civic Orchestra, the training orchestra for the world renowned Chicago Symphony Orchestra. After high school, Marie studied writing at Columbia College in Chicago, Illinois.

Marie lives in Lombard, Illinois with her husband Steve and their daughter Evelyn. They share their home with their dogs Honey and April, and their cats Fairfield and Neptune.

Marie is currently recording a solo cello CD called *Orange on Blue* which will be released in spring 2008. She is also touring with her unforgettable performance *Weaving: an Inspirational Journey*.

For information about booking *Weaving: An Inspirational Journey* for your organization, please contact Marie through her website: www.maries-cello.com or send her an e-mail: sirbarclay@maries-cello.com